MAXIMIZE
YOUR
METABOLISM

MAXIMIZE
YOUR
METABOLISM

LIFELONG SOLUTIONS to LOSE WEIGHT,
RESTORE ENERGY, and PREVENT DISEASE

NOEL MACLAREN, MD
SUNITA SINGH MACLAREN

WITH RECIPES FROM VIVIAN CIOFFI

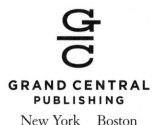

GRAND CENTRAL
PUBLISHING

New York   Boston

Copyright © 2021 by Sunita Singh Maclaren and Noel Maclaren

Cover design by High Design. Cover image by Getty Images. Cover copyright © 2021 by Hachette Book Group, Inc.

Grand Central Publishing
Hachette Book Group
1290 Avenue of the Americas, New York, NY 10104
grandcentralpublishing.com
twitter.com/grandcentralpub

First Edition: April 2021

Grand Central Publishing is a division of Hachette Book Group, Inc. The Grand Central Publishing name and logo is a trademark of Hachette Book Group, Inc.

The publisher is not responsible for websites (or their content) that are not owned by the publisher.

The Hachette Speakers Bureau provides a wide range of authors for speaking events. To find out more, go to www.hachettespeakersbureau.com or call (866) 376-6591.

LCCN: 2020949422

ISBNs: 978-1-5387-1882-7 (hardcover), 978-1-5387-1881-0 (ebook)

Printed in the United States of America

LSC-C

Printing 1, 2021

For Manjit Kirpal Singh,

a beloved mother who,
for over four decades, has courageously shown
that your genes need not be your destiny

CONTENTS

PART III
The Protocol

INTRODUCTION

The scientific spirit does not rest content with applying that which is already known, but is a restless spirit, ever pressing forward towards the regions of the unknown.

—Archibald Garrod, *Inborn Errors of Metabolism*

On a molten August late afternoon in the MetaKura Clinic waiting room, Luisa, thirty-six, an executive assistant at a multimedia conglomerate, fanned herself fervently with a magazine. Her mahogany hair was gathered in a topknot. Seated across from her, Noam, fifty-seven, a jovial self-confessed workaholic in the jewelry business, with brown fawn-like eyes, dabbed his moist forehead. Suddenly, Colby, a slender, ginger-bearded twenty-three-year-old, entered the waiting room and sat down. His head thrown back, he quickly appeared to drift into a languorous nap, but then began drooling. Perspiring profusely, he slumped forward. We all congregated around him, trying to slip glucose tablets under his tongue. Colby became nonresponsive; his eyes firmly closed. An eerie stillness clung to his inert body.

"Well, we know he's alive because I can hear him snoring gently," pronounced the nurse who had been cajoling Colby to sip orange juice. Within minutes, a tangerine-vested emergency medical crew placed an intravenous drip into the young man's arm. Colby stirred; his blood glucose levels were now restored. We collectively exhaled and resumed breathing normally. It turns out that because Colby's body had long since stopped making insulin naturally, he had taken an injection of it to manage his type 1 diabetes.

The hormone insulin may be thought of as a stealth messenger that stimulates glucose in the blood to enter into muscle and fat cells in the body to create and store energy. Because Colby was in a rush and had forgotten to eat his lunch, as his blood glucose level declined, his brain began to malfunction. Colby is normally *insulin sensitive*, meaning that his body's cells are quick to respond to the hormone's signals to promptly regulate glucose levels in the blood within a narrow range.* As Colby's glucose-deprived brain began to falter, it resulted in his hypoglycemic (low blood sugar) crisis.

Luisa is *insulin insensitive,* meaning that her body cells are genetically predisposed to a more lethargic response to the hormone, resulting in higher blood glucose levels and more insulin needed for vital metabolic functions. C-peptide lab tests, which measure circulating insulin levels in the body, show Luisa's resting levels of the hormone to be as much as three times as high as Colby's at the time of his emergency. At first glance, Luisa's body appears to have adapted brilliantly to compensate for this aberration, enabling her to regularly run ultramarathons. But if you look more closely, another picture emerges. Even with all her running, Luisa has not been able to shake off her excess weight nor her foggy spells of depression.

In the case of Noam, who has type 2 diabetes, his pancreatic islet cells have to generate six times the normal amount of insulin to help him get through his twelve-hour workday. Noam's body's impaired response is called *insulin resistance.*

Consider the following statement to be one of the Ten Commandments of Biology. "All the [body's] vital mechanisms, varied as they are, have only one object, that of preserving constant the conditions of life in the internal environment." It was made by a vintner's son and onetime vaudeville playwright, who later discovered a passion for medicine. Born in the village of St. Julien-en-Beaujolais, Claude Bernard (1813–1878)

---

* Between 4.0 and 5.4 mmol/L (72 to 99 mg/dL) when fasting and up to 7.8 mmol/L (140 mg/dL) two hours after food

was recognized in his lifetime as one of the giants of science. Bernard created the notion of the *milieu interieur*. His observation about the need of complex organisms to regulate a stable internal environment in the face of a subzero climate, a viral pandemic, or a heart-pounding two-hour dance led to neurologist and physiologist Walter Cannon coining the term *homeostasis*.[1]

Insulin is the primary controller of energy homeostasis in the human body. As it permeates the variegated landscape of virtually every type of human cell, its range of actions is exquisitely regulated and highly differentiated between bodily organs. When insulin resistance causes signaling defects and clutters the intracellular pathways in the body and the brain, the effects are compellingly wide-ranging.

For nearly 800 million years, insulin, this pearly-chained hormone—the simultaneously most studied and most mysterious molecule in medicine—and its precursors enabled living organisms to store energy for times of food scarcity or for sudden energy needs.[2] Insulin resistance is an evolutionary form of energy conservation that enabled our Paleolithic hunter-gatherer ancestors to survive periods of food deprivation by signaling the body to store fat instead of burning glucose as energy. In our post-Neolithic age of nutritional plenty, adverse stress patterns, deficient exercise, and reduced sleep, this inherited genetic adaptation, which affects one in four people, has resulted in a range of metabolic imbalances so the body appears to have gone rogue. We, like others in the medical profession, daily witness this shift that represents a fundamental and growing change in human health as habitual insensitivity to insulin is passed from one generation to another.

There is an added twist to this picture. In 1971, Tibor Gánti, a Hungarian biochemist and author of *The Principles of Life,* observed that our body's regulatory mechanisms depend on an internal-external gathering of clues, "the metabolism is a unit of life; it is inherently stable, it contains an informational subsystem and it is regulated and controlled." In this instance, a genetic adaptation for survival has created the possibility that the body's tightly controlled glycemic control system can be bypassed.

Externally, culture (lifestyle choice) is the enabler both for exacerbating the symptoms of insulin-signaling defects but importantly also offers pathways for its correction. Our patients did not realize that because of their diminished response to a domineering hormone, a steady diet of Luisa's favorite Sicilian vermicelli pasta and Noam's ancestral Jewish Mashhadi cuisine served with basmati rice would progressively change their appetite signals and increase their hunger patterns. More seriously, they did not fully appreciate that these glucose-elevating foods would make them more vulnerable to brain fog and depression.

MAPPING THE METABOLISM

Every second, hundreds and thousands of reactions occur within a cell to provide life-giving energy—collectively known as the metabolism or the command center of human performance capabilities. So powerful is this complex messaging system that its telltale imprints can be found in every cell and organ of the human body. As we will show in the chapters that follow, the full range of the metabolism is thrown off kilter when insulin, its paramount messenger, goes into overdrive. Our survival is driven by twin needs, described by the Russian writer Ivan Turgenev thusly: "Love and hunger share the same purpose—life must never cease; life must be sustained and must create."

Your metabolism profoundly affects your energy levels, cognition, moods, body shape, and size. It also plays a major role in your sex hormones, sleep, likelihood for muscle pain, and ability to absorb essential nutrients. Additionally, it factors into your risk for cardiovascular or psychiatric disorders—and can increase your chance of succumbing to a virus. The telltale hallmarks of defective insulin levels can cause disarray in all these spheres of human health.

While scientists do not fully understand all the mechanisms that have contributed to the rise of this increasingly prevalent metabolic imbalance, we can evaluate a range of clues. Early signs of its appearance include excess body weight and reduced fertility. We know that a pregnant mother's habits affect her unborn child for life. During periods of neonatal distress, genes receive "tags" or instructions for their deactivation, which change their function but not their structure. The Dutch *Hongerwinter* (famine) of 1944 to 1945, the Great Chinese Famine from 1958 to 1961, and the food shortage in Biafra, Nigeria, from 1968 to 1970 all resulted in children of low birth weight, below what is expected for their gestational period. Paradoxically, as adults these individuals disproportionately struggled with excess weight and, in some instances, hypertension and type 2 diabetes.[3]

At our MetaKura Clinic, we find that a convincing majority of our patients who are insulin resistant were born prematurely or had a low birth weight based on their gestational period. Average body weight is on an upward trajectory the world over, and heavier women, as well as their babies, are more likely to be insulin resistant during pregnancy. Fetal insulin regulates intrauterine growth, and when the hormone's signals are blunted, babies are born one or two pounds smaller than expected for their gestational age. This was the case with both Luisa and Noam, whose inadvertent choices in their daily regimens triggered their range of symptoms for a metabolism in distress. In our clinic experience, a minority of babies who are born large for their gestational age go on to exhibit eating disorders in later life. Our results and those of others show that with modest lifestyle adjustments, sensitivity to insulin, this commanding presence among body messengers, is linked to weight loss and improved body fat distribution.[4]

We hold that insulin resistance is an inherited type of metabolic profile that is lifelong and one that has been programmed by birth. Despite this genetic hardwiring, the outcome is dependent on the choices that are made in diet, exercise, sleep, stress, and other areas, which is our reason for offering this book to you. The immensely good news is that by making lifestyle choices and changes as we have seen in thousands of patients at the MetaKura Clinic, the health complications associated with this silent blood sugar dysfunction are preventable and sometimes *reversible*.

Crucially—and here is where we believe that our work breaks new ground—we have found that most adverse insulin resistance patterns can be permanently improved within six months.

ONE IN FOUR

Each person's molecular profile, their unique metabolic signature, can be captured in a moment in time by a lab analysis that measures huddles of fats and proteins in the body. These biomarkers, or indicators of a risk for illness, are constantly changing. One unruly biomarker can change the pattern of the others. But it doesn't have to. As you'll learn, with each unwelcome change in a person's metabolism come *mutatis mutandis*—changing the things that need to be changed—which is an opportunity for its correction. Our goal with this book is to capture the MetaKura Clinic's comprehensive expertise—medical, lifestyle, behavioral, nutritional, and fitness—for you to be able to maximize the full potential of your own metabolism.

With the discovery of new biomarkers and aided with artificial intelligence–enabled wearable technologies, it is now possible to offer highly personalized solutions to regulating health outcomes. We can make fairly accurate predictions about a person's longevity based on their genes and other biomarkers, their diet, and their exercise patterns. But even without these molecular analyses, you can follow the steps that we have outlined in this book to better understand and take charge of correcting your metabolism.

For one in four people with insulin resistance, the intricate physiological architecture of their metabolism has, to varying degrees, gone astray. These types of metabolic personalities are implicated as the primary cause for type 2 diabetes and Alzheimer's, both of which are expected to grow in global prevalence by about fifty percent in the next thirty years.[5,6] Expectant mothers with gestational diabetes are more likely to have a child with autism, which is also dramatically on the rise.[7] This dysregulation of insulin in the body reveals itself with a constellation of distressing symptoms: dark circles around the eyes, recurring fatigue, lingering depression or anxiety, urgent food cravings, low fertility, and a propensity for stockpiling body fat, among others. In addition to a tendency to store body fat, other features of chronically elevated levels of insulin include chronic myalgia (muscle pain and aches), a deflated libido, triglyceride dysfunction, and a greater risk for cardiovascular disease and strokes. A blunting effect on the muscle glucose transporter GLUT4 makes it harder for glucose to enter muscle cells, often leading to chronic tiredness, which, counterintuitively, can be corrected with exercise. Less well known is what we like to call the Frida Kahlo effect, the higher levels of androgenic, or male-like, hormones that we have seen in countless female patients.

Chances are, you can find symptoms of insulin resistance in your own family tree. We certainly can: A chubby, restless artist father who succumbed to a stroke in his fifties while researching Goya in Madrid. A jovial uncle, a celebrated military general who began to fade with Alzheimer's. A disapproving aunt with a whisper of a mustache. A moody cousin who once lapsed into clinical depression. And Sunita's mother, Manjit, dressed in her silks and artfully matched jewelry, who carries an insulin syringe in her sequined evening bags. Miraculously, by carefully following the regimen designed for her, Manjit has managed to keep her glucose levels mostly within the normal range for forty-four years.

The heroes of our book are our patients who have endured the disruption of their hormones with remarkable courage and dignity. And, most important, the majority have been willing to make the necessary adjustments to become the primary champions of their own well-being, brain health, and longevity.

Noel Maclaren

When I think about my academic and clinical practice careers, I find that the peptide hormone insulin has played a central role. As a high school senior in New Zealand, I narrowed my career choices to geology or medicine. I eventually chose the latter option, perhaps because of my

Presbyterian upbringing; I wanted to have a livelihood that would help people. During my first hospital residency rotation in internal medicine, I encountered a musically gifted woman in her late twenties who was blind, had no sensation in her feet, and was in renal failure because of her diabetes. She dutifully followed all of the medical advice given to her, but we, the medical profession, had clearly failed her. I began to think that I would like to discover better medical solutions for people like her and embarked on a career as an adult endocrinologist. Eventually, I moved to London, where I also became certified in the pediatric area of my specialty.

As my career progressed, at Johns Hopkins School of Medicine, I, along with my able colleagues, began studies to investigate the suggestion by the late Dr. Lawson Wilkins that type 1 diabetes was an immunological disease. Our research quickly concluded that he was right.[8,9] My further research at the University of Florida amplified support for this idea.[10,11] We went on to show that using antibody markers, family members at risk could be identified long before the onset of type 1 diabetes, and we could screen people in the general population.[12,13] This led to promising therapies for its prevention.[14]

Later, while at Cornell, my colleagues and I observed that women affected by polycystic ovarian syndrome (PCOS) were prone to developing type 2 diabetes. Through my roles as an endocrinologist caring for children, pregnant women, and other adults, I came to understand that insulin resistance is a common genetic disorder affecting about one in four persons, with an outcome that depends upon their lifestyle choices.[15] I was all too familiar with the subtle effects of insulin and began to design comprehensive new methods of predicting and reversing the effect of insulin resistance. Working with my wife, Sunita, the solutions we devise for our patients are culturally based with small but permanent lifestyle modifications so that they can be readily adapted to their lives.

Sunita Singh Maclaren

When I came to live in the United States more than thirty years ago, I resolved to try to contribute to my new hometown of Houston, Texas. My small advisory firm, which later moved to New York, designed highly tailored cultural solutions for the global challenges faced by governmental agencies, corporations, and nonprofits. These included customizing global leadership programs that we taught in parts of West Africa, Southeast Asia, and the Russian Far East based on the histories of local communities, and assessing new cross-border products and services for their cultural suitability. Aside from these projects and our global engagements with U.S. government agencies and the International Criminal Court in The Hague, we also worked extensively in healthcare and medical anthropology.

Whether we believe in Western, holistic, or other forms of medicine, our sense of our physical well-being is interpreted through our cultural filters. Healing, then, is a subtle, nuanced conversation between biology and culture. It is integral to every society and can take many forms. For example, on the walls of the Musée du quai Branly—Jacques Chirac museum of anthropology in Paris—are hundreds of masks, amulets, and charms from across the spectrum of human history and geography that were fashioned to ward off ill health.

Our firm's fieldwork showed the explosive effect of cultural practices on underlying genetic predispositions for insulin resistance. Rice, maize, wheat, combined with sorghum, tubers such as potatoes, cassava, yams, and taro are the staples of global ethnic cuisines, which uphold a shared sense of national identity for 7 billion people in the world. Yet these foods cause a steady rise in blood sugars, which, especially for people with insulin resistance, are increasingly being linked to accelerating cognitive decline.[16] In adults, it is widely acknowledged that those with type 2 diabetes are especially prone to suffer alterations in brain function and structure, although we do not fully understand the underlying mechanism.[17] Social rituals like late dinners (popular in Madrid, Mumbai, and Buenos Aires) and shortened sleep (customary in Tokyo and Seoul) interfere with the release of hormones like growth hormone (GH), melatonin, cortisol, testosterone, and prolactin, which are highly regulated by our sleep-wake cycle. Over two decades, my gifted colleagues and I worked on projects in cities and remote locations in thirty countries, including Kuala Lumpur, Argentina, and Papua, Indonesia, among many others. I soon realized that I had an affinity for those who felt a sense of otherness and that I enjoyed working with people to help resolve complex problems with knowledge-based programs.

I made frequent visits to BioSeek Clinics, Noel's full-service endocrinology clinic in Manhattan, and became increasingly spellbound by the insulin-resistant patients I met. Their eyes shone as they recounted stories of their personal transformations. They were relieved to have found a name for their seemingly unrelated, maddening symptoms. Under Noel's resourceful care, by making changes to their diet, these patients had joyfully reclaimed a sense of well-being and, as a side benefit, lost much of their unwanted body weight (or were in the process of doing so). In 2011, Noel and I decided to collaborate professionally, and we launched MetaKura (*kura* is the Maori word for wisdom), a clinic-cum–innovation lab for people with insulin resistance. A team of committed dietitians and fitness experts joined us to provide ongoing support to our patients. Soon we began suggesting modest adjustments in our patients' daily sleep, exercise, and relaxation rituals, in order to add new layers of solutions that would help to stabilize their insulin levels. The cumulative effect of this approach, our patients told us, was a jolt of new energy and a noticeable improvement in their cognition and mental clarity.

People with inborn errors of the metabolism often feel misunderstood. They are unfairly blamed for their excess weight when the root cause is primarily genetic. Another reason we began the MetaKura program is because our patients' stories of the prejudice that they encounter in their everyday life reminded us of the people who have been subjected to stigma because of their ethnicity, religion, or gender. Our goal is to support people who come to our clinic when society has chosen to discredit them for no good reason.

After guiding hundreds of people on their six-month journey of metabolism correction and weight loss, all the while questioning them closely about their life patterns, we have learned to recognize these "personalities" from afar. These collective impressions led us to design a questionnaire for determining a metabolism personality. Each type has different dietary, exercise, and sleep needs from the others. From the outset, we understood that in order for our solutions to be sustainable over a lifetime, they had to be personalized to be effective, and they had to be easy in order to be readily accommodated into people's lives.

Our New York City location means that our patients represent a dazzling montage of humanity. They include Black opera singers, New Jersey mothers, Brazilian bankers, Orthodox rabbis, Brooklyn schoolteachers, Puerto Rican software designers, and teenagers from Greenwich, Connecticut, among many others. Each has their own behavioral cues, dietary preferences, and varied routines, which are, in the words of the anthropologist Clifford Geertz, "spun in a web of [cultural] significance."[18]

Our multidisciplinary approach involves an investigation of clues both from medicine and human behavior. In 1848, the physician-anthropologist Rudolf Virchow wrote, "The task of science is to stake out the limits of the knowable, and to center consciousness within them." Once we diagnose insulin resistance, our goal is to help the individual identify the dietary, social, and behavioral adjustments they should make to keep it well under control. Our patients must enact these changes for life, and it doesn't take long for them to see why. They are quick to tell us of the unhappy consequences they suffer when they stray from the MetaKura program, but because their goals are for the long term, we stress that they must forgive themselves for occasional lapses—because regaining control of their insulin and metabolism is for life.

INSULIN AND ITS EXCESSES

"Action!" "Easy does it!" "Switch off!" Cells take their orders from a cascade of tiny, potent signaling molecules. Unlike neurons or the immune system's T-cells, which are the body's two other interdependent messaging networks, hormones such as insulin can be precisely measured. There is a mathematical precision to how the body's messenger hormones—which are quantified in nanograms, picograms, and femtograms, or one thousand billionth of a gram—work together in a way that we find similar to solving sudoku puzzles. There is an inherent, almost musical logic to the orderly and correct placement of the numbers.

In evolutionary terms, 400 million years separate humans from jawless hagfishes (Myxiniformes). Yet the protein structure of that ancient creature's insulin sequence of amino acids is 61 percent similar to that of humans. This constancy over millennia of the long pearly chain that forms insulin's structure highlights the hormone's vital role in all living creatures. Insulin signals can be observed in the tiny earth roundworm, *Caenorhabditis elegans*, which has an average life span of a mere twenty days. Salmon, bovine, and porcine insulin were once extracted for human therapies. Why is insulin, described as "the secret quintessence of life" so vital? Insulin's job is to break down our food, enabling our cells to obtain glucose for energy. We cannot survive without glucose because it fuels energy production in mammalian cells, especially the brain. Next to breathing, our survival depends upon a tight regulation of our glucose levels made possible by a sophisticated cascade of signaling responses between our vital organs, as well as adipose (fat) and muscle tissue.

THE METAKURA MASTER PLAN

Our solution is offered in three simple steps: diagnosis, prevention or correction, and lifelong maintenance. In lieu of the biomarker tests that we conduct in our clinic, we have designed the Metabolism Self-Assessment Questionnaire (see page 31). This assessment mirrors the questions that we would ask our patients in an initial clinic consultation. Once you have completed the assessment, your responses will lead you to one of four metabolism personality types: Jade, Sapphire, Emerald, or Ruby. These types are based on insights that we have gained from over twenty years of working with thousands of patients.

Part II of the book, "Elements of the Metabolic Matrix," provides a guide to our solutions. It explains in detail, based on your metabolism personality, the ten elements of the Metabolic Matrix, all of which represent opportunities where you can intervene to improve your longevity, cognition, and sense of well-being. Pieces of this intricate jigsaw puzzle of metabolism are especially relevant for people with insulin resistance. Each chapter, which represents a separate element of a matrix, will allow you to explore the different interlocking jigsaw pieces that influence your metabolism and look for themes and patterns that may be most relevant for you.

Part III, which is focused on nutrition, offers lifelong practical suggestions for enhancing your metabolism with fresh, easy, and delicious recipes from a talented chef, a patient who joined our program and became a dear friend, Vivian Cioffi.

As with any beguiling puzzle, challenges and mysteries remain in unraveling the secrets of the intercellular processes that occur within organisms to maintain life. We have devised many solutions. Let's begin solving the mystery of you.

PART I

Your Metabolism Personality Type

CHAPTER 1

The Metabolic Matrix

Energy is eternal delight.
—William Blake

Our focus is on a phenomenon that we believe should take center stage as a key determinant for improving your cognitive capabilities, health, and longevity—if you have an inherent bodily resistance to insulin and its complications. In each chapter of *Maximize Your Metabolism*, you will encounter popular myths, breathtaking scientific and cultural leaps of insight, and the essential knowledge in that field that we have found most clinically useful. We hope to enable you to mastermind your own metabolism.

Our concept of a "matrix" has little in common with the 1999 science fiction action film. Instead, if we go back in time to the early Latin era, the meaning of "matrix" was derived from *mater* (mother)—a source of life, an embodiment of nature, a force that supports and sustains. In 1850, a British mathematical genius, J. J. Sylvester, used "matrix" to refer to a rectangular sequencing of numbers which he said "offered unlimited possibilities."[1] We favor both uses of the word.

Your unique metabolism is at the core of who you are. It shapes your identity, your perceptions of the external world, your susceptibility to disease, and strongly influences the full range of your human capabilities in every stage of your life. Yet it is not entirely fixed. Instead, your metabolism is more akin to a kaleidoscope, one that is capable of startling changes. The matrix we have designed is based on the principle of creating harmony with each interdependent element. Use it to identify any adverse factors that pertain to you, as well as to find the necessary remedies. As with any complex calculation, a successful approach to overcoming a challenge is one that assesses all the unique contributing factors and then corrects them one by one. While we wish we could meet you face-to-face and offer individual biomarker tests and the personal consultations we provide at the MetaKura Clinic, we are pleased to share what we have found to be most helpful to our clients—albeit in a somewhat simplified form.

It is important to understand that while the modifications that we suggest are proven to be highly effective, they should be adopted gradually and become permanent. Extreme diets or drastic lifestyle changes, when introduced suddenly, are rarely successful in the long term, so we do not recommend them.

ELEMENTS OF THE METABOLIC MATRIX

Your biology, your personal and family medical history, as well as your patterns of nutrition, exercise, and sleep contribute to far-reaching cascading cellular effects inside you, which all come into play in creating your personal metabolism profile. You will learn here how each of the elements of the Metabolic Matrix influences your health in more detail in future chapters, but here are some highlights on their powerful influences. Your metabolism profile will be your guide as to the best approaches for you to master each element and enable you to design your own blueprint to maximize your health, well-being, and longevity.

Genetic Legacy

Insulin resistance is strongly familial. Despite advances in the sequencing of the human genome, there are only rare instances of structural gene mutations to explain it.

We believe that the more likely cause is epigenetic, meaning environmental influences that permanently change gene expression. Genes can become dynamic interpreters of our interactions with the environment, and their functions can be disabled (imprinted). The epigenome is the collection of "tags" that can turn genes on or off. For many of the 25 percent of the global population whose biological, cognitive, and emotional well-being is altered by insulin resistance, such epigenetic changes have become heritable, meaning that they can be passed on to children and grandchildren.

Madrid's Prado Museum counts among its most well-known works the portrait of Eugenia Martínez Vallejo, a six-year-old girl dressed in yards of red brocade who was born with an uncontrollable appetite. Painted in 1680 by Juan Carreño de Miranda, the court painter for Charles II, the girl in the painting has now become a torchbearer for young people with Prader-Willi syndrome, a rare metabolic disorder. She is reassuring proof to those diagnosed with the condition that their excess weight is caused by their genes and not by their behavior.

Nutritional Profile: Food, Culture, and Identity

Nutritional responses to the same food vary from person to person. As a Sapphire, Emerald, or Ruby personality, you have a metabolism that will be overpowered when you eat simple carbohydrates. For people like you, this category of food—which includes fructose, sucrose (sugar and sugar alcohols), grains, and starches—will not only result in increased bodily fat stores but will also affect your moods and fertility patterns.

The MetaKura Protocol favors foods that uplift various aspects of the metabolism, including complex carbohydrates like buckwheat and beans, which improve appetite signals and digestion.

We especially encourage clients to consume prebiotic foods that enrich a varied internal garden of gut bacteria (our microbiome).

"Changing my diet has improved my cognition," said Gayle, one of our patients. "Earlier I may have had to read a paragraph three times. Now I can read pages of data and retain it. And that's pretty cool."

Hunger: Signals That Fine-Tune the Appetite

- **Brain**—The hypothalamus stimulates hunger, as well as the feeling of satiety. It is important to allow time for the brain to register fullness after food intake. Satiety is induced by chewing food, so in our view, which is supported by scientific data, juiced foods bypass the signaling that indicates feelings of fullness, resulting in higher calorie intake.[2]
- **Gut**—Following a healthy meal or snack, the digestive tract has multiple gatekeepers that set off alerts to signal fullness. Commercially prepared foods are designed to override and distort our body's built-in hunger modifiers. We recommend complex natural foods, eaten at a leisurely pace that stimulate the gastrointestinal satiety hormones.
- **Fat cells**—As surely as a hammer finds a nail, an increase in body fat changes a person's appetite signals. Leptin is a satiety hormone produced by adipocytes or fat cells when the stomach fills. Insulin dysregulation makes the brain less responsive to leptin,[3] and it also affects another metabolic regulating hormone, adiponectin. This means that you can develop the habit of eating past the point of appropriate satiety.

Gut Reaction: The Power of the Microbiome

Antioxidant foods like raspberries and cabbage reduce the presence of food-derived cytokines—a family of proteins that is associated with inflammation, pain, and aging.[4]

The digestive benefits of inulin, found in the chicory root coffee of New Orleans, have been recorded in early civilizations. It is mentioned in the Ebers Papyrus of ancient Egypt, and written texts of Greeks and Romans, including Aristophanes and Horatius, recount descriptions of chicory eaten roasted or raw.[5] Today it is a popular salad ingredient in Belgium, France, and the Netherlands.

Fat Cells: Exquisitely Designed Hubs of Energy?

A key issue for physicians treating metabolic disorders is managing high triglyceride levels, which contribute to liver damage and hardening of the arteries, which in turn increases the risk for strokes and heart attacks. High triglyceride levels can be corrected with dietary modifications that reduce consumption of carbohydrates, *not fat*. To minimize risks for heart attacks and strokes, we also pay close attention to other lipid irregularities like low levels of protective high-density lipoproteins (HDL), or good cholesterol, that removes other lipids from your blood stream.

Although it is often vilified, cholesterol deserves our gratitude. It comprises a major part of the structure of the brain and retina in the eye. It endows all animal cell membranes with life-giving fluidity and permeability. This commonly dread-inducing member of the lipid family is essential for the creation of vitamin D, adrenal hormones, and sex steroid hormones. Fat cells trigger chemical reactions involved in growth, immune function, reproduction, and other aspects of basic metabolism. Above all, the circle of life, the core of our means of survival, is accomplished by storing and activating fats, our energy reserves.

Energy: Speed, Strength, Movement

Contrary to popular belief, people who carry excess body weight have a higher overall energy expenditure because it takes more energy to support a larger body mass. Significant weight loss over a short amount of time predisposes a person to rebound weight gain, especially because successful dieters tend to have permanently low resting energy expenditures.

Prolonged exercise increases insulin sensitivity. Regular, repetitive fitness routines increase the presence of muscle cell glucose transporter (GLUT4), thereby bringing more oxygen and nutrients to the muscle tissue.

It's never too late to start. Late-blooming athletes should be inspired to know that studies have shown that there was no difference in starting age between higher skilled and lesser skilled athletes. Additionally, physical fitness, but not the level of physical activity, was associated with improved cognitive function, specifically with those areas of brain function related to language ability, attention, and processing speed. Motor skill acquisition leads to procedural learning, which can be retained for long periods of time.

Enhancing Cognition: Thoughts, Moods, and Memory

With aging, the brain progressively loses its capacity to metabolize glucose, especially in those who are insulin resistant. There is a stronger association between poor glycemic control (seen with type 2 diabetes) and a loss of memory, poorer executive control, and processing speed in the brain.

Paul Ehrlich, a German bacteriologist and Nobel laureate, in 1908 discovered that water-soluble dye, when injected in the bloodstream, did not penetrate the brain. The blood-brain barrier tightly controls the movement of molecules, ions, and cells between the blood and the central nervous system. Recently, magnified brain imagining has shown that leaks in the blood-brain barrier associated with metabolic dysfunctions like diabetes and insulin resistance are prevalent in people with Alzheimer's, depression, and bipolar disorder.[6]

Countering Stress: Cultivating Mental Resilience

Cortisol, a steroid hormone, is essential for life, supporting as it does our cardiac and immune capabilities. The physiological stress response leads to the release of cortisol from the adrenal glands, which increases energy availability in the short term. Chronic stress interferes with insulin signaling at a cellular level. Importantly, it increases the level of glucose in the blood. Bioscience research has repeatedly confirmed a direct correlation between higher blood glucose and cortisol levels in accelerating the onset of diabetes.

Venturing far from the Anglo-Saxon world lie timeless treasures and stratagems in cognitive restructuring. For example, between 500 and 200 BCE, the Indian sage Patanjali presented the goal of yoga (*chitta vritti nirodha*) as "the easing of mental fluctuations."

In 1925, the psychiatrist William Sadler referred to "Americanitis" (a term that he borrowed from the psychologist William James) as "a result of the tension, the incessant drive of American life, the excited strain of the American temperament."

Sleep: Circadian Rhythm and Blues

The French astronomer and physicist Jean-Jacques d'Ortous de Mairan observed in 1729 that mimosa plants unfurl their leaves in sunlight and curl them up at night. Even when placed in a darkened space for several days, the plants continued to follow this diurnal pattern. He surmised that the plants were controlled by an internal mechanism now known as the circadian clock.

Habitual sleep deprivation leads to a classic three-dimensional portrait of insulin resistance: chronic fatigue and weight gain often accompanied by depression. Poor quality or short sleep (less than seven hours on average) leads to lower glycemic control. During REM sleep, vital hormones are released for bodily restoration while cognition is promoted through dreaming.

Irregular breathing patterns, or sleep apnea, are found in up to 77 percent of overweight men and about half as many women in the same category.[7] In our experience, sleep apnea treated with respiratory aids can be reversed with appreciable weight loss.

Hormone Imbalances: A Few Cases of False Alarms

A prolonged volatility of insulin levels also suppresses the actions of the body's hormone transporter proteins called serpins (serine protease inhibitors). As a result, isolated measurements of certain hormones do not reflect their actual functional levels.[8] This commonly leads to incorrect lab readings of low thyroid hormones or low testosterone, as we will explain more fully in Chapter 12.

Serpins regulate stress, sexuality, energy, heart rate, and circulation. They are involved in a range of bodily processes, including the transmission of nerve impulses and transport of hormones.

Finally, we believe that our clinic patients' impressive outcomes can be attributed to the simple dictum of the Renaissance philosopher Francis Bacon, namely *scientia potentia est,* or knowledge is power. When someone arrives for a medical appointment armed with a scrawl of questions and sheaves of pages printed off the internet, we warm to them. Their curiosity and enthusiasm for probing the hidden secrets of their physique will, in our experience, lead them to become formidable champions of their own well-being.

The MetaKura program is based on clinical proof that as you explore the essential knowledge of the elements of the Metabolic Matrix and fine-tune your insulin levels, your mental and physical well-being will grow by leaps and bounds. As you learn how the ten elements of the matrix work together, how they affect you, you can repeatedly redesign your own matrix, in a manner that is uniquely beneficial to you.

CHAPTER 2

Your Metabolism's Personality

The book of nature is a fine and large piece of tapestry rolled up, which we are not able to see all at once, but must be content to wait for the discovery of its beauty, and symmetry, little by little, as it gradually comes to be more and more unfolded, or displayed.

—Robert Boyle, Anglo-Irish physicist and inventor (1627–1691)

Arthur Conan Doyle, the polymath physician-author, once wrote that in creating Sherlock Holmes he wanted a "scientific detective who solves cases on his own merit and not through the folly of the criminal." The practice of endocrinology necessitates the skills of a sleuth who uncovers hidden clues, often in unexpected places. For the purposes of this book, we are presenting four simple typologies of metabolism profiles—Jade, Sapphire, Emerald, Ruby—that are viewed through the lens of the degree to which insulin is exquisitely regulated by vital organs of the human anatomy. We have developed these profiles to help our patients with metabolic ailments—90 percent of those without diabetes are unaware that the root cause of their combination of distressing physiological, emotional, and cognitive symptoms is insulin insensitivity.

For fifteen years, the MetaKura Clinic has devised ways to moderate insulin-related surges in the body and thereby to reverse or minimize its ensuing complications. Having successfully treated thousands of people, we feel confident that these four personalities represent a workable spectrum of this vastly undiagnosed metabolic imbalance. Our Jade, Sapphire, Emerald, and Ruby personalities have been developed to help you identify the concrete steps you or your older family members can take to improve your metabolism at whichever stage you are, and to prevent or reverse its associated complications.

Our methodology is well represented in Claude Bernard's classic work *An Introduction to the Study of Experimental Medicine*, where he wrote, "Medicine is but a part of human biology and [also] the study of human inheritance, constitution, intelligence and behavior, of adaptation to new conditions of life, and of a host of other subjects, [all of which] far transcend the boundaries of medicine."[1]

HOMO "HYPER INSULIN" SAPIENS

At the MetaKura Clinic, more often than not, an insulin insensitive personality is instantly recognizable, long before their confirmatory lab reports are obtained. These individuals tend to have hairlines receding at the temples, thinning hair or, in women, facial hair. They may have adult acne. High levels of testosterone in women, a side effect of these hormonal excesses, cause these symptoms.

At our practice, together with a careful scrutiny of a person's biomarkers found in their bodily fluids that assess their susceptibility to a disease, we emphasize narrative medicine. By this, we mean a detailed account of the person's medical conditions and those of their family members. Oliver Sacks, neurologist and best-selling author, called this "the interface of biography and biology." Susceptibility arising from our personal histories, those of our parents, siblings, and grandparents, are all embedded in our genome, where some genes are expressed, and others are silenced.

We know that over time, the brain becomes insulin resistant. Starting in the forties, the stability of brain networks begins to decline, although these effects can be delayed with dietary changes.[2] Not uncommonly, patients with unregulated hyperinsulemia (excess insulin) are dogged by anxiety from early childhood and, later, by memory loss. As stated earlier, there is convincing evidence that mothers with gestational diabetes are three times more likely to have children with autism.[3] Unwanted body weight also makes mischief in accelerating depression and anxiety and vice versa. An astonishing 80 percent of people with Alzheimer's have insulin resistance and/or type 2 diabetes. One of the first improvements our clients observe on the MetaKura program is greater mental clarity and a boost in their cheerfulness and sense of optimism.

A CHANGEOVER

Elliot, age sixty-two, owner of a recruitment agency for software engineers, requested an urgent clinic appointment. As we went over his family history, his breezy, self-assured manner briefly cracked, and his voice suddenly grew hoarse: "My younger son is twenty-five years old. He just had a stroke and we almost lost him." Elliot's salt-and-pepper-haired wife, who is also his business partner, squeezed his hand as he continued. "I've come to clean up my act, Doc. My father always said, hasty climbers have sudden falls. I hope you can help me."

Clinic Notes

Elliot's extensive tests presented a picture of a man on the edge of a cliff. At five foot five, he weighed 272 pounds and had a body mass index (BMI) of 43.5 (a BMI of 30 in men is associated with a shortened life span). Elliot's BMI* was at a level where it can interfere with basic physical functions such as breathing or walking. His mother had died of a stroke at sixty-five years of age, and his twin sister had diabetes. His

---

* Body mass index (BMI) is a person's weight in kilograms divided by the square of their height in meters. A high BMI can be an indicator of high body fatness. The National Institutes of Health designates BMI of 27.3 in women and 27.8 in men to be overweight and a BMI of 30 in either sex to be obese. A simple BMI calculator can be found on the NIH's website: https://www.nhlbi.nih.gov/health/educational /lose_wt/BMI/bmicalc.htm.

father, a robust ninety-five-year-old retired theater producer, lived on his own on the Upper West Side of Manhattan. Elliot's blood sugar was at a hazardous level (HbA1c* 12.3 percent), placing him at a high mortality risk; he was at least one hundred pounds overweight, and his lipid profile (triglycerides) were seven times the upper end of the normal range. On his first physical exam, dark discoloration (*acanthosis*) was observed on Elliot's eyelids and neck, a sign of elevated levels of insulin.

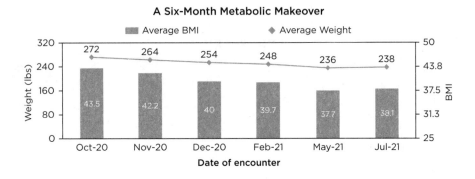

A Six-Month Metabolic Makeover

Test	Initial	After 6 months
Blood sugar (HbA1c)	12.2%	5.2% (diabetes ≤5.7%)
Triglyceride	718	83 (normal ≤140)
Liver enzymes	50	14 (normal ≤35)

Miraculously, six months after joining the MetaKura program, Elliot brought all his vital health indicators nearly within a normal range and had lost his first thirty-four pounds. As a bonus, he was able to negotiate far more favorable terms on his life insurance policy.

---

* A hemoglobin A1c (HbA1c) test measures glucose levels in the blood.

DIFFERENCES ARE MORE THAN SKIN DEEP

Each person's metabolism is a unique combination of billions of cells that regulate their internal environment and are in turn subject to countless external factors, notably lifestyle decisions. Within the same family, individuals who share similar genetic susceptibilities, dietary habits, and life patterns can display a significant difference in the expression of the personality and character of their metabolism. When the Bellucci family boarded a ship to New York from the Campagna region near Naples, Italy, in 1972, Sofia, a shy sixteen-year-old, was accompanied by her boisterous, dark-haired sister, Rita. Neither spoke any English. Although five years apart in age, they have the preternatural bond of identical twins. By their mid-twenties, the sisters had married a pair of brothers. When Sofia qualified as a schoolteacher in Queens, Rita chose the same profession. Now, Sofia, sixty-five, and Rita, sixty, are grandmothers, and the three generations of Bellucci family bonds are a marvel to behold. Initially, they contacted the clinic about a newborn family member born with a rare thyroid disorder. Within a few months, five Bellucci family members became our clinic patients. All four Bellucci women share a genetic legacy—as do 25 percent of the rest of the world's people—of a flawed energy metabolism called insulin resistance, which manifested differently in each member of the family. Rita and Sofia—together with Rita's two adult daughters, Carina and Alessa—joined the MetaKura program. All followed a similar meal plan that we designed for them. At the end of six months, their results were as different, as the Italians say, *come il giorno e la notte,* as night and day.

In that time, Sofia lost forty-seven pounds, thirty pounds more than her relatives. Rita, known as the night-prowling family insomniac, began sleeping through the night. Her older daughter, Carina, found that her pervasive anxiety and brain fog—"I'm the speech therapist who could not recall words," she joked—had lifted. Alessa, the baby of the family and now a mother of three, said, "Earlier, my hunger controlled me. Now I control my hunger."

THE METAKURA METABOLISM PERSONALITIES

We have devised four archetypal metabolism personalities, keeping in mind that there are countless variations within each category. Each personality, named for one of four timeless gems, represents a progression from a simple to a more complex profile of the imbalances in the metabolism caused by wayward insulin levels. Within each category, every gem, like each one of you, has a distinct personality. Each gem metabolism personality has its own meal, exercise, and sleep plan, which is based on the degree to which you or your loved ones display symptoms associated with a breakdown of cellular insulin communication. Making dietary changes alone—based on the metabolism personality you will soon identify based on our questionnaire—will greatly assist you in improving and maintaining your health and mental acuity.

Jade Metabolism Personality Profile

Sapphire Metabolism Personality Profile

Emerald Metabolism Personality Profile

Ruby Metabolism Personality Profile

Our metabolism personality profiles are as follows:

Jade personalities are *not* likely to be insulin resistant, but there are gratifying steps they can take to master their metabolic health and improve their insulin sensitivity.

 Sapphire personalities, likely as a result of family history, have a real risk for insulin resistance, although they appear to be asymptomatic. They can make dietary and other corrections in their habits now to avoid future complications.

 Emerald personalities have begun to show overt symptoms of hyperinsulemia. These changes can be reversed, and Emeralds can stop the advance of these symptoms before they reach a stage of disease complications.

 Ruby personalities have medical complications from their insulin resistance. Fear not, however, because they will, in all likelihood, immediately feel revived after making a few changes in their daily rituals and food choices.

METAKURA METABOLISM SELF-ASSESSMENT QUESTIONNAIRE

© Copyright MetaKura 2020

Please circle the boxes that apply to you and total the score. If you are not sure of the answer, skip to the next question rather than trying to guess. The more accurate your answers, the more personalized your results will be. After you have completed all parts of the questionnaire, your total score will indicate which personality you are.

Part One: Your Physical Features

	yes	no
Were you born prematurely?	1	0
If no, was your birth weight between 7 and 9 lbs.?	0	0
If no, was your birth weight more than 9 lbs.?	1	0

(continue)

Part One: Your Physical Features *(continue)*

If yes, was your birth weight 6.5–7 lbs.?	1	0
If yes, was your birth weight below 6.5 lbs.?	2	0
Do you consider yourself to be overweight?	1	0
Is your present body mass index (BMI) less than 25?	0	0
Is your present body mass index (BMI) 25–30?	1	0
Is your present body mass index (BMI) 30–35?	2	0
Is your present body mass index (BMI) over 35?	3	0
Do you have stretch marks/ striae on your skin? (women, before pregnancy)	2	0
Do you have adult acne?	2	0
Do you have hair loss around your temples?	2	0
Do you have skin tags on your face, neck, or underarms?	2	0
Do you have dark patches on your neck, underarms, and/or around your eyes?	2	0
Women: Do you have unwanted facial hair?	1	0

Part One Score:

Part Two: Your Inherited Family Risk Profile

Family Member	Type 2 Diabetes	Clinically Overweight BMI 30+	Hypertension (High Blood Pressure)	Gout	Alzheimer's Disease	Polycystic Ovarian Syndrome (PCOS) (women)	Total Score
Father	2	1	2	1	1		
Mother	2	1	2	1	1	1	
Sister 1	2	1	2	1	1	1	
Sister 2	2	1	2	1	1	1	
Brother 1	2	1	1	1	1		
Brother 2	2	1	1	1	1		
Aunt	1	1	1	1	1	1	

Uncle	1	1	1	1	1	
Grandma	0.5	0.5	0.5	0.5	0.5	0.5
Grandpa	0.5	0.5	0.5	0.5	0.5	0.5
Part Two Score:						

Part Three: Your Personal Health Profile
Have you been diagnosed with any of the following conditions?

	yes	no	score
High blood pressure	2	0	
Type 2 diabetes?	2	0	
Do you take insulin?	1	2	
Is your diabetes once controlled without insulin?	2	0	
Do you take pills to manage your diabetes?	2	0	
Were you diagnosed with diabetes after 35 years of age?	2	1	
Have you had bariatric surgery?	2	0	
High blood sugar (but not diabetes)	2	0	
Low HDL cholesterol	2	0	
High triglycerides	2	0	
Numbness in your feet	1	0	
Pancreatitis	2	0	
Gallstones	2	0	
Sleep apnea (interrupted breathing during sleep)	2	0	
Gout	2	0	
Women only: Polycystic ovarian syndrome (PCOS)?	2	0	
Women only: Have you had gestational diabetes?	2	0	
Part Three Score:			
Total Score from Parts One, Two, and Three:			

Your Metabolism Personality	
Jade Metabolism Personality	5 points
Sapphire Metabolism Personality	5–10 points
Emerald Metabolism Personality	10–15 points
Ruby Metabolism Personality	15+ points

Physical Features of Sapphire, Emerald, and Ruby Metabolism Personalities

Those who are insulin resistant may have:

- Dark circles around the eyes, and dark pigmentation on the lower eyelids, underarms, and neck (*acanthosis nigricans*)
- Facial hair in women
- Adult acne
- Hair loss in men and women
- Skin tags on the face and neck
- Stretch marks (striae) on the trunk or thighs
- Excess weight in the abdomen or hip areas
- Missed menstrual periods

Other common symptoms:

- Chronic fatigue, anxiety, or depression
- Poor sleep patterns
- Difficulty with weight loss
- Brain fog or difficulty concentrating for long periods

Jade Metabolism Personality

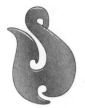 The Aztecs and Mayans considered jade to be the most precious of stones. Confucius called jade the jewel of heaven. The Chinese, who revere the stone for its quality of immortality, refer to the highest Daoist divinity, the Jade Emperor (known as Yu Huang), as the ruler of heaven and earth. Even today, it is believed that jade is protective because it helps balance the body's fluids and promotes harmony and well-being.

Jades are at the lowest risk for insulin resistance and therefore have the least possibility for its medical complications. The most definitive proof of this is of course a lab test. Whether by design or sheer luck, if you fit this metabolism personality, your choice of nutrition and hours of sleep and exercise are, so far, working in your favor. There is much you can do to fine-tune your metabolism if and when problems arise. Jades should be proactive about their health, especially when overweight or underweight or if they experience anxiety or chronic fatigue.

Jades may be less aware of the sugars hidden in foods, snacks, and drinks. Dietary ignorance may lead to unwanted weight. Some Jades eat excessive amounts of food for pleasure (hedonic eating) without awareness of the potential harm from it. You may also sleep too little, exercise inadequately, be overly stressed, and lack regular means of relaxation. Of the above concerns, eating habits loom large but are readily correctable.

Family History

Jades may themselves be moderately overweight, but they tend not to have a family history of diabetes or strokes. Unlike other personalities, Jade's family lineage does not appear to include metabolic imbalances like gout, high triglycerides, hypertension, and Alzheimer's. In addition, Jade's birth weight tends to be within the normal range for the length of the gestation period.

Physical Features

Body mass index, known as your BMI, is a measure of fat based on height and weight in adult men and women. A majority of Jades have a BMI of 18.5 to 25.0. For some Jades, your lifestyle choices may have put you outside of this range. If you are an athlete, pay special attention to our section on energy and movement (see Chapter 8) to improve your performance capabilities. For the Jade personality profile recommended food list and metabolism guidelines, see page 221.

Margaret

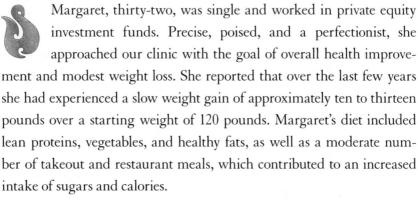

Margaret, thirty-two, was single and worked in private equity investment funds. Precise, poised, and a perfectionist, she approached our clinic with the goal of overall health improvement and modest weight loss. She reported that over the last few years she had experienced a slow weight gain of approximately ten to thirteen pounds over a starting weight of 120 pounds. Margaret's diet included lean proteins, vegetables, and healthy fats, as well as a moderate number of takeout and restaurant meals, which contributed to an increased intake of sugars and calories.

She had periods of anxiety as a child. Originally from Ohio, Margaret had come to the New York area for her MBA and immediately following her graduation found work that she loved. She tended to skip breakfast, eat a late dinner, minimize her sleep during the week, and drink two or more glasses of Chardonnay to help her relax in the evenings. Childhood anxiety can change the eloquent dialogue between the nervous and endocrine stress response system, commonly known as the hypothalamic pituitary adrenal (HPA) axis. Among the changes we suggested to Margaret was to make a high-protein and fiber breakfast part of her daily routine. We also advised her to carefully read all food labels to ensure that no food that she ate had more than five grams of sugar or simple carbohydrates per serving. Margaret began to opt for dry martinis instead of cocktail mixers and for red over white wines as the former have less sugar, as well as to limit herself to one drink per day with food. Because her weight-loss goals were modest, Margaret's consumption of complex carbohydrates was less restricted, though complex carbohydrate dietary choices were encouraged. Margaret added Pilates and kickboxing classes as part of her weekly exercise routine. She also adopted a puppy for companionship to help her relax after work.

Margaret worked long hours, and we suggested that she keep a high-fiber snack at her office. Within four months, she lost eight pounds. She slipped briefly, adding a pound or two when her parents came to stay with her in New York for two weeks and she pampered them with delectable, although not always metabolism-friendly, meals. Six and a half months after she began the MetaKura program, Margaret was down to 122 pounds, and her digestion, sleep patterns, energy, and *joie de vivre* had improved.

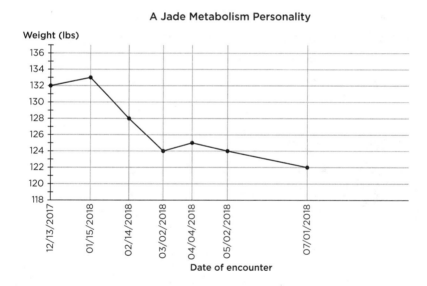

A Jade Metabolism Personality

Alan

Alan was a twenty-one-year-old computer analyst who reported fatigue, loss of libido, and weight loss. His general practitioner had referred him to us because his testosterone level was extremely low, at 20 ng/ml where normal is 350 to 1,100 ng/ml. After some hesitation, Alan admitted to having carefully restricted his diet to shed unwelcome extra pounds that he had accumulated over the winter months. An ardent vegan, he had reduced his food intake to 650 calories a day—as part of that frugal diet he somewhat obsessively ate exactly sixteen hazelnuts every day—and in so doing, he had lost thirty-five pounds. Indeed, when we first saw him, his BMI was only 16.5—well below the 18.0 threshold for being underweight. After much discussion, Alan agreed to increase his food consumption (we advised 2,000 to 2,200 calories per day) and he gained twenty pounds, giving him a BMI of 20.5. This led his testosterone level to rebound to near 500 ng/ml and with it, his symptoms resolved. In Alan's case, severe food restriction had lowered the level of a fat-cell hormone (leptin), which in turn disabled the ability of the brain's hypothalamic region to regulate sex hormones. The cumulative effect was to nearly halt his body's secretion of testosterone. This is an extreme example of the consequences of an overly restrictive diet. Nutritional balance is an important key to health.

Jades, by studying the Metabolic Matrix carefully and creating a fresh, new blueprint for yourself, you can be confident of your ability to enjoy robust health now that will carry you into your later years.

The Sapphire Metabolism

Sapphire has been prized as a great gemstone since 800 BCE. Known as the "wisdom stone," the sapphire is a symbol of power and strength, but also of kindness and wisdom. Ancient rulers believed that the color of the sky was a reflection of sapphire stones. In medieval times, sapphires were believed to offer protection from poison, plague, and fever. Under Pope Innocent II, senior clergy wore sapphire rings to demonstrate their connection to divinity. Sapphires are worn by some to restore balance in the body and to release mental stress.

If you are a Sapphire, you should be aware that, based on your responses to our questionnaire, you likely have inherited metabolic imbalances associated with insulin resistance, although you may not yet show any symptoms. This may result in cravings for comfort food, a sense of chronic fatigue, or periods of brain fogginess. You may also feel that you are losing your battle against adding extra girth to your waist. These symptoms are not a reflection of your poor lifestyle choice, but rather that your body is programmed to favor weight gain and may be adversely affected by your dietary choices. Sapphire, we want to stress the importance of your being proactive from this moment on. One of the most far-reaching risks with chronically elevated levels of insulin is cognitive decline. You have the opportunity to avoid a long-term pattern of weight gain and detrimental health complications.

Sapphires may share certain physical features with the Emerald and Ruby profiles. However, because your risk level is more moderate than Emeralds and Rubies, you have fewer restrictions on the simple carbohydrates in your diet and a less intense minimum requirement for exercise. You can now make the choice to be a Sapphire for the rest of your days and minimize your health risks.

For a Sapphire personality food and metabolism plan, see page 223.

Helen

Tall and attractive, Helen has a commanding presence with her stylish outfits accented with Native American turquoise jewelry. On her first visit to the clinic, this fast-paced fashion editor, known to be a ball of fire, uncharacteristically burst into tears. Her body felt slow, heavy, and unresponsive to her choice of diet. "My assistant, who organizes my meals, says that I barely eat a thousand calories per day," she said after noting her body weight of 203 pounds. "And yet I just keep feeling that my clothes don't fit!"

Helen was the primary income earner for her family of four. Her work diary was crammed with international travel and client entertainment. Because she often had no control of how her meals were prepared, her daily diet was closely monitored by our dietitian. Helen, predominantly vegetarian, occasionally also ate fish and eggs. To improve Helen's metabolism, we addressed her vitamin D deficiency and designed a meal plan that reduced her overactive appetite signals (see Chapter 5). After

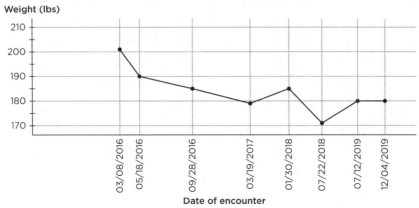

A Sapphire Metabolism Personality

Weight (lbs)

Date of encounter

four months on the diet we prescribed, Helen said that she felt that her body was working better; meanwhile her dress size had dropped from size 14 to size 10. In six months, Helen was thrilled to have her husband and her colleagues compliment her on her new look as she lost a total of twenty-eight pounds. More importantly, she said, her ability to concentrate for long periods had improved, as had her overall sense of contentment. She had a brief setback nine months later, regaining three pounds after enjoying a few too many desserts while on vacation.

Once she understood the genetic trajectory of insulin resistance, Helen became alert to her eight-year-old son's growing tendency for chubbiness. Sure enough, laboratory testing revealed that he also had indications of insulin resistance. As of this writing four years later, Helen feels in control. She exercises five times a week, and has lost thirty-six pounds altogether. She and her son continue to do well.

The Emerald Metabolism

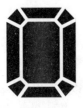

In Hindu philosophy, the emerald heart chakra ensures physical, emotional, and mental equilibrium. Worshipped by the Incas and favored by Aristotle, Alexander, and Cleopatra, emeralds are said to inspire deeper inner knowledge, a quality we most wish for you. Emeralds are worn for harmony in love and friendships.

If you are Emerald, your metabolism is already showing signs of distress. Based on your responses to the questionnaire, you have probably inherited genes that cause your body to be progressively less sensitive to insulin. Chronically high insulin levels are beginning to cause undesirable complications for your long-term body and brain health. Emerald, you stand at the crossroads of a life of robust good health and energy, or one of increased risk for medical complications. Act now! We are here to help you. The good news is that by making a few permanent changes in your diet and lifestyle, you can reverse any effects of metabolic distress, like an enlarged liver or excessive abdominal fat. Your metabolism, like your brain's neuroplasticity, is highly adaptable. Step into the driver's seat and take charge.

Emeralds may share certain physical features with Sapphires and Rubies as they all have the same genetic predisposition to insulin resistance. Because their metabolism has been showing more symptoms than a Sapphire personality, but they have not yet reached the point of medical complications like Rubies, Emeralds will have to be vigilant with creating a plan for themselves that covers all ten segments of the Metabolic Matrix. Your goal should be to use the knowledge provided here to change your profile to a Sapphire metabolism in six months' time.

Family History for a Sapphire and Emerald Metabolism

If you have a parent or sibling with diabetes or if you had a birth weight that was lower than expected by one or two pounds, chances are that you have inherited genes that will make your body less sensitive to the hormone insulin. Over time, insulin resistance (IR) can put you at risk for type 2 diabetes, high blood pressure, liver dysfunction, and even Alzheimer's. Moreover, if you have a chubby child who started life as a low birth weight baby and there is a family history of diabetes, he or she is also at risk.

For an Emerald personality food and metabolism plan, see page 226.

Ezra

Ezra's father owned a popular electronics store in Manhattan. His mother, petite and well-spoken, blazed a trail in the real estate business. Yet in Ezra's Orthodox Jewish neighborhood, people shook their heads sadly when they talked of his family. At twenty-six, Ezra weighed 320 pounds, took antidepressants, and stayed at home because he had not been able to keep a job. At night, his parents said, it was as if swarms of locusts had invaded their kitchen. Cabinet doors were left ajar, snack wrappings littered the floor, anthills of bread crumbs covered the counters, and dirty plates filled the kitchen sink. Ezra's appetite was out of his control. His parents resolved to take action, and on the recommendation of a member of their synagogue, who himself had been a successful client on the MetaKura program as a Ruby personality, they brought Ezra to the clinic.

The vital connection between food choices and mood and cognition is an emerging field called neuro-nutrition. Ezra and thousands of others like him with insulin resistance tend to find simple carbohydrates irresistible, indeed addictive. Unfortunately, these are the foods that create the highest insulin responses in the body. Prolonged elevations in insulin lead to glucose depletion in the muscles, resulting in chronic fatigue. Faced with ongoing tiredness, people like Ezra curtail their activities and gradually withdraw into themselves, a common symptom for depression. Almost without exception, people on the MetaKura program remark upon a newfound sense of mental energy once they eliminate a few harmful foods from their diet and begin to exercise more.

The first step was to create a tailored meal plan for Ezra that would not only accommodate his kosher diet but would also be compatible with his long commute to New Jersey for an accounting course in which he had recently enrolled. Ezra's parents were initially unconvinced that the MetaKura program would work. On the first day, for example, he ate an entire supersized bag of almonds that were recommended as part of his diet, all in one go. However, with continuous support and

An Emerald Metabolism Personality

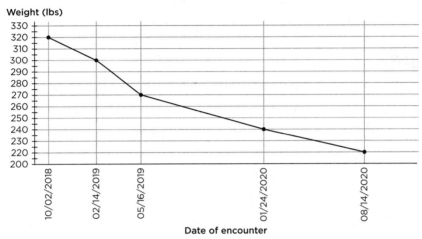

encouragement, Ezra settled into his new regimen and slowly began to feel less hungry. He was also noticeably more upbeat and energetic. Soon neighbors began telling him that he looked more fit.

This was the first time in a long while that Ezra had felt successful, and that sense of accomplishment spilled over to other areas in his life. His nightly visits to the gym became sacrosanct. Six months after joining the program and minus forty-five pounds, Ezra made a triumphant visit to see his cousins in Israel. As of this writing, he has lost ninety-nine pounds and works a full-time job at a nursing home. Every so often, his proud parents send us photos of a handsome, athletic man with a gleeful smile who is on the lookout for a bride.

The Ruby Metabolism

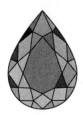

The earliest residents of ancient Babylon believed that star rubies offered protection from ill health. Sanskrit scriptures refer to rubies as *ratnaraj,* or "the emperor of jewels." Many cultures associate the ruby's bloodred hue with passion, protection, and prosperity.

If you fit in the Ruby profile, you have advanced levels of insulin resistance, which have resulted in medical complications. Rubies may have insulin resistance genes from multiple sources in their family tree. Perhaps you are taking medication for type 2 diabetes, hypertension, gout, or liver complications. If so, we recommend that you discuss any changes in your diet, lifestyle, or medications with your medical practitioner or endocrinologist. The lifestyle interventions and dietary adjustments suggested for the Ruby profile will improve the effectiveness of medications you may be taking or in many cases could actually reduce or eliminate the need for them. Again, this step should only be taken in consultation with a physician.

The good news is that by making a few permanent changes to your diet and lifestyle to complement any medication that you may have been prescribed by your doctor, there is much that you can do to improve your health and potentially reverse your metabolic complications. If you are currently a Ruby personality, it is possible to transform yourself to an Emerald or Sapphire personality—think of it as a form of metabolic alchemy.

Family History

Rubies may have inherited insulin-related complications, either on both sides of the family or possibly more strongly prevalent among their maternal or paternal relatives. Another possibility is that a Ruby personality has excess weight that has led to medical complications.

Other Medical Complications

Ruby personalities may have one or more of the following complications:

- Obesity or morbid obesity
- Type 2 diabetes
- Hypertension
- Dyslipidemia
- Fatty liver disease
- Gallstones
- Pancreatitis

- Gout
- Atherosclerotic heart disease
- Sleep apnea
- An increased risk of common cancers
- Alzheimer's

Ruby personalities may also be more prone to:

- Anxiety, chronic fatigue, and cognitive impairment
- Depression
- Issues with sleep
- Issues with fertility for women

For a Ruby personality food and metabolism plan, see page 229.

Pamela

 Pamela, forty-three, announced with dread on her first visit to the clinic, "My grandfather and great-grandmother had their legs amputated [due to diabetes], as did my grandmother Lula, who was a grand old Southern lady." Despite her daily workouts and closely monitoring her diet, Pamela had recently been diagnosed with diabetes. She felt devastated not to have escaped this part of her family heritage.

A Yale-trained lawyer, Pamela led her firm's legal strategy that resulted in the company winning a $30 million lawsuit in Paris. She said, "My grandparents on both sides came from sharecropper families in Jim Crow country in the Mississippi Delta. My happiest childhood memories are of my summers in my mother's hometown. There were big, wide-open spaces, and the sense of freedom was amazing." Her grandfather, she explains, was a respected member of the community and owned 150 acres of land. "My mother picked cotton till her twenties. Five generations of family members lived together." Pamela kept a promise that she had made to her single mother, from when she was an eleven-year-old girl, and got a full scholarship to university. By the age of twenty-four, she was a practicing lawyer.

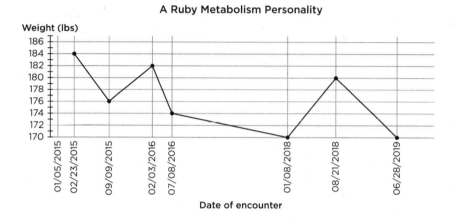

A Ruby Metabolism Personality

Then she added ruefully, "For the last twenty years, I have been putting on and losing the same twenty pounds. I spent six months on assignment in Europe and made myself miserable to lose eight pounds. I had two weeks at home, and even though I was very careful, all I had lost came right back on."

After joining the MetaKura program, Pamela found relaxation in a new avocation. "I was always interested in quilting because it was a long-standing family tradition. My grandmothers, great-grandmothers, and others were talented quilters. Quilting gives me an escape and forces my brain to work in a completely different way. I love the combination of the precision, creativity, and skill."

Clinic Notes

Pamela's concern about her own risk for complications from diabetes was appropriate. She inherited the insulin resistance gene shared among many of her relatives. Her sister, mother, maternal grandfather, and all six maternal aunts and uncles shared the same medical diagnosis. She understood that she had inherited disease-prone genes rather than her health issues being solely a result of her lifestyle. Only drastic changes in food choices and daily habits could lower her own medical liability in the future.

Because Pamela joined the MetaKura program primarily to reverse her symptoms of diabetes, our dietitian was instructed to design a meal plan that emphasized lean proteins, high fiber, no grains or sugar sources, and frequent small meals. She began following a fitness routine in the gym four days a week, worked out with a trainer once a week, did yoga, and tried to walk a couple of miles every day. Pamela looks younger and happier, having stabilized her blood sugars (HbA1c from 7.1 to 6.5 percent), lost fifteen pounds, and has devised ways to follow her dietary regimen wherever she happens to be. Most of all, she (and we) is confident that with these changes she can avoid ever having to take insulin.

Finally, remember that by finely calibrating your metabolism, you can enhance your appearance, your moods, your energy levels, your mental clarity, and reduce your risk for health complications. In Part II, you will obtain a deeper understanding of managing the key elements that control your distinct physiology so you can experience a new sense of all-around satisfaction with your life.

Elements of the Metabolic Matrix

CHAPTER 3

Genetic Legacy: The Mischievous Messengers Lurking in Family Trees

We do know that there is a basic genetically-built architecture in the body which really, to a large extent, determines our resistance, or susceptibility [to weight gain]. Excess weight is one of the strongest genetically influenced states we have.

—Dr. Stephen O'Rahilly and I. Sadaf Farooqi, Cambridge University[1]

When people come to the MetaKura Clinic, they almost always experience a singular moment, often accompanied by tears, when they learn that their distressing symptoms of unwanted body weight, erratic sleep patterns, and disabling fatigue are *not* primarily the result of unfavorable lifestyle choices. Rather, the primary cause is in the genes that they have inherited, genes that have been altered by the environment or ones that may have gone silent across generations of a family. In this chapter, we explain the reasons for these DNA deceptions in metabolism and why they have grown exponentially in recent years, to the point that one in four people worldwide is now affected. Nonetheless, as you will learn, you can change the course of your genetic destiny.

The first consultation at our clinic begins with a detailed investigation of the individual's metabolism-related medical history, as well as that of their close blood relatives: parents, grandparents, siblings, aunts, and uncles. In almost every case, genetic patterns reveal themselves fairly quickly. This suggests a phenomenon that is termed *genetic dominance with variable penetrance*. Penetrance refers to the proportion of individuals within a family, each with a genetic propensity for a certain trait, who also actually exhibit that trait. We then follow up, where necessary, with clinically relevant lab tests that include genetic markers.

A VORACIOUS APPETITE

Tall and burly, Ariana's father, Patrick, still has the mullet haircut that is a giveaway of his earlier life as a drummer in a rock band that played gigs in the eighties at New York City's famed CBGB. When he signed the deed on a three-story brick home in Marine Park, Brooklyn, in 1995, Patrick embraced the neighborhood's civic motto, *Improve, Don't Move*. He continues to reside in Brooklyn but now lives alone. First, he lost his wife, Madelaine, to breast cancer, and recently he admitted his teenage daughter, Ariana, to a special hospital program in Pennsylvania. She weighed 398 pounds.

From infancy, Ariana's appetite grew more voracious by the day. By age eleven, she would take food off people's plates and grab fistfuls of dog biscuits at Petco. "Five years ago, when Madelaine was in the late stages of cancer," Patrick said, "she would cry that she was leaving behind a thirteen-year-old daughter who would never have a normal life. 'God doesn't love me,' Madelaine would lament."

Patrick explained the current challenges. "While playing with a puppy last summer, Ariana broke her ankle. Once she was immobilized, the weight just accumulated until she reached almost four hundred pounds. Now she's at a special hospital in Pittsburgh, where she will remain for at least two months, on a diet of six hundred calories a day. She lost twenty pounds in the first two weeks. She's really happy there and enjoys the company of the other teenagers. Like any seventeen-year-old, she dreams of having a boyfriend." Father and daughter are now active members of a support group for Ariana's rare inherited metabolic disorder.

Clinic Notes

When we first saw Ariana as a six-year-old, she weighed 110 pounds. She had low muscle tone, tapered fingers, and a drooping lower lip, which are all classic symptoms of Prader-Willi syndrome. This appetite disorder, which also affects cognition and pubertal growth, is estimated to affect one in every fifteen thousand people. People with Prader-Willi have an uncontrollable appetite because the hypothalamic area of their brain receives a hormonal hunger signal from the stomach regardless of whether the person has just eaten or not. The satiety centers in the brain of an individual with Prader-Willi cannot feel the signal of fullness that normally occurs after eating a meal. Most people with this condition have elevated levels of the hunger-inducing hormone ghrelin, as the body tries valiantly—but unsuccessfully—to communicate satiety to the brain.[2]

In Ariana's case, our clinic-initiated DNA tests showed that her father's protective Prader-Willi syndrome gene, while normal, was switched off—what is called imprinting—confirming the clinical diagnosis of this rare condition. As is the case in all people, the Prader-Willi gene inherited from the mother is silent, so it was unable to help Ariana. But here's a compelling fact: contrary to the popular association of excess weight with diabetes, despite once weighing close to four hundred pounds, Ariana was not insulin resistant; nor did she have type 2 diabetes.

Instead, Ariana's appetite-signaling genes were locked into an "off" position as the result of a gene-silencing chemical process called DNA methylation. People with her condition also have challenges with fertility, which explains why the condition is rare.

Prader-Willi is uncommon. But what happens when such changes in *other* metabolism-related genes, like insulin resistance, are family wide, multigenerational, or influenced by the environment?

Himsworth's Hindsight[3]

Harold (Harry) Himsworth headed the UK Medical Research Council from 1949 to 1968. A Yorkshire boy who briefly worked at a worsted mill to help support his family, Himsworth kept such a low profile at University College Hospital that examiners had to send for his official photograph to identify him when he won the first of two University Gold Medals in 1929. As a professor there, Himsworth had a scientific insight that was forty years ahead of its time. After studying the results of an experiment conducted in 1936 where patients were given a glucose drink, a shot of insulin, and a blood test, Himsworth was the first to observe that people had two types of reactions. Those he called *insulin sensitive* patients customarily showed acute symptoms of urination, hunger, and thirst in childhood (type 1 diabetes) and could tolerate a generous intake of carbohydrates with minimal doses of insulin required to keep their urine free from traces of sugar. The rest—those in whom higher doses of insulin had minimal effect—he called *insulin insensitive* or *insulin resistant*. The insulin-resistant patients, whose symptoms were more subtle and surreptitious (type 2 diabetes), passed sugar in their urine after consuming small portions of carbohydrates.

"Research being an enquiry into the secrets of nature, the condition for its effective prosecution is an undivided attention to the phenomena of the natural events under study. Human needs or wishes are, in this context, aberrations. It is essentially a voyage of discovery," said Himsworth. John Lister at the Royal Free Hospital in London began using blue and white cards to identify his patients as having type 1 or type 2 diabetes using Himsworth's frame of reference.

In 1977, in her Nobel lecture, the New York-based medical physicist Rosalyn Yalow described insulin as "the principal regulator of fat metabolism."

A National Institutes of Health study shed light on the coordinated cellular responses in insulin-insensitive cells that lead to excess body weight. Glucose, obtained from food, provides cells with a wallop of energy. Within nanoseconds of glucose being released into the bloodstream, the pancreas dispatches insulin to alert the muscle and fat cells to take in glucose. In fat cells, as soon as the insulin molecule docks into its cell receptor, a cascade of signals beckons glucose transporter proteins (GLUT4) to appear at the cell's surface to ferry glucose inside the cell. Using high-resolution imaging and a fluorescent dye, the researchers observed that in neutral liquid, individual molecules of GLUT4 in a fat cell were evenly distributed across the cell membrane. But when exposed to high levels of insulin, as would be the case for people with insulin resistance, the rate of total GLUT4 entry into the fat cell membrane peaked, quadrupling within three minutes—sixty times more often on fat cells exposed to insulin than on cells not exposed to insulin.[4]

TAMARA'S DISPLACED ANCESTORS

"We were so steeped in our Ukrainian world that even though I was born in Silver Springs, Maryland, I spoke English with an accent," says Tamara, a thirty-four-year-old nurse who has an Emerald metabolism. Her parents represent the third wave of Ukrainian migrations, arriving in New York in 1955 and 1956, after living in a camp for displaced persons in the medieval town of Mittenwald, Germany.

"We call ourselves DPers—displaced persons—because we have grown up in the shadow of our parents' traumatic dislocation," Tamara explains. "Mentally, my parents and their whole generation were harking back to their homeland. My sisters and I went to a Ukrainian Saturday school, attended evening socials at a Ukrainian church, and spent our summers in camps for Ukrainian kids in upstate New York."

Tamara's father was a shy but brilliant man with a drawer full of Mensa honors his family discovered after his death. Tamara says, "Dad was the parent we turned to when we had boyfriend problems. He and my grandfather were great storytellers, and both struggled mightily with their weight.

"I, like them, was always the fat kid who could not fit into my sisters' hand-me-downs. The neighbors would call me *pampushky*, the puffy donuts filled with poppy seeds, or *bubliki*, an East European bagel. They would say, 'There is so much of you to love,' or 'You must be the one who spends time in the kitchen with your mother.' Later at nursing school in Baltimore, I'd make myself walk for miles and miles. But I noticed that while my classmates could eat two hamburgers late at night and remain stick thin, my waist expanded even as I dined only on salads."

Now Tamara lives in Brooklyn with her husband and two daughters. Marina, her younger daughter, was born two years after her sister, Julia. Marina was the smaller infant at birth. Tamara says, "When the family sits down for the same meal, Julia can eat three times more than her sister and still look like a twig. Marina and I aren't like that. However, I don't want to shame her the way my mother inadvertently did with me.

"I remember picking up Marina at school and seeing her lined up with the other students and thinking that I needed to stop letting her eat donuts. But when I heard from Marina's teacher that she was skipping gym, using the excuse that she could not open her locker, I decided it was time to bring her to your clinic."

Clinic Notes

Tamara's paternal grandfather must have been insulin resistant (IR), which he passed down to his son, who passed it on to her. Little Marina also tested positive for the condition, establishing that the real cause of her weight gain was that she had inherited her mother's metabolic phenotype. Marina's birth weight was lower than that of her sister, Julia, the initial sign, also seen in premature babies, that she might be insulin resistant. Fortunately, Tamara understands the genetics of this disorder and does not blame her younger daughter for her weight, as her own mother once blamed her.

Tamara could see how easily Marina gained weight even as she ate far less than her lean sister, Julia, who inherited her father's insulin sensitive genes. The degree of insulin resistance can vary depending on its prevalence in the maternal and paternal family trees. When we instructed the family to eat a low-carbohydrate diet, Marina lost weight decisively, albeit slowly. A parent who has made good lifestyle choices may not show features or complications of insulin resistance but nonetheless pass that gene on to a child, who does exhibit these signs. This heritable mode of transmission is a dominant trait, in which the chances of any child inheriting the trait is akin to a heads-versus-tails coin toss. In this case, one daughter inherited her mother's insulin resistance and the other did not.

HOW GENES IMPACT HEALTH

Not all the metabolic attributes you get from genes lead to health problems, nor are they subject to being influenced by your lifestyle or environment. Heritability refers to variations in a trait such as height or dimples that result from genetic rather than environmental factors. The heritability of height is believed to be 0.80 to 0.85.[5] This means that 80 to 85 percent of the differences in height in a select group of people may be attributed to genetic variances within that group. In other words, if a woman is six feet tall in a community where the average height is five foot ten, 80 percent of her extra height may be attributed to her genes and the remaining 20 percent to nutrition and other environmental factors. Between 1914 and 2014, eighteen-year-old women in South Korea averaged a gain in height of 7.84 inches.[6] So genes are the primary factor, but regular exercise, healthy foods, and other lifestyle choices also play decisive roles in the outcomes of those genes. Similarly, studies on the heritability of body mass index have been measured at 0.78 and waist circumference at 0.76, respectively.[7] However, when comparing identical pairs of twins with nonidentical (fraternal) twins, the genetic effect explained body size by up to 70 percent.[8] As with height, a person's body size and the idiosyncrasies of their metabolism are highly influenced by their underlying genetics. Alexander Graham Bell and his father, Melville Bell, both died of complications of diabetes. Elvis Presley's mother, Gladys, died at just forty-six years old of heart disease and a compromised liver, both hallmarks of underlying insulin elevations that had not been addressed adequately. Elvis died even younger, at forty-two, weighing 350 pounds and having been diagnosed with type 2 diabetes.

"From now on, Dad, we are going to have a very different conversation," declared one young woman when she discovered that she had inherited her parent's genes for insulin resistance. Her father, a senior partner in a Wall Street brokerage firm, had joined the MetaKura program to address his wayward lipid profile and return to the body weight he had as a twenty-five-year-old. He succeeded. His bright-eyed, canny thirteen-year-old daughter was forty pounds heavier than her twin brother, who had been spared this genetic susceptibility. The insulin resistance she had inherited was primarily responsible for her propensity for nocturnal food cravings. An inherited tendency for this type of metabolic distress does, however, need enablers from the environment.

Untangling Genes and the Environment

Epigenetics looks at the interplay between genetic inheritance and the environment. It encompasses the study of chemical modifications that occur to genes at different times and that influence gene activation. An oft-cited analogy posits that if the genome is an orchestra, epigenetic regulation represents the conductor's notations on the sheet music that will determine the manner in which the orchestra's musicians will play their respective instruments. Epigenetics, a term coined by the embryologist Conrad Waddington in 1942, is the study of gene regulation independent of DNA sequence. Epigenetic processes play a role in the regulation of all biological traits from conception until the end of life. Breast cancers have been linked to epigenetic changes in gene expression.[9] Epigenetic therapies, used to reverse gene mutations, are now offered as treatment for a form of leukemia.[10]

After World War II, the research community began to explore whether extreme stress could affect the expression of genes and might explain the heritability of excess weight. This inquiry had a historical source: when the Germans occupied Holland, they imposed severe food restriction on the entire population in retaliation against resistance groups that had derailed Nazi trains. This led to the severe *Hongerwinter* (hunger winter) of 1944 to 1945, which caused more than 20,000 deaths from starvation. Official daily rations in Holland ebbed from 1,800 calories per day in December 1943 to 1,400 per day in October 1944. At its worst moments from December 1944 to April 1945, daily rations ranged from 400 to 800 calories, causing an estimated 18,000 deaths from starvation. Said one survivor, "It was an awful, terrible time—people were scraping [garbage] bin lids with spoons, they were so desperate."

A remarkable study by nutritionist and biochemist Dr. Elsie Widdowson and her colleague Dr. Robert A. McCance, which was later confirmed by others, found that babies born to mothers who experienced the starvation period in their first trimester of pregnancy exhibited increased rates of diabetes, hypertension, and excess weight as adults. However, if the starvation period occurred in the second or third trimesters, the infants did not experience greater rates of any of these three conditions as they grew and developed.[11]

Neonatal Programming

It is now well established that low birth weight based on the gestational period is a predictive sign of insulin resistance. Dr. David J. Barker, a genial-faced, snowy-haired English physician and epidemiologist, was described by longtime colleague Dr. Kent Thornburg as having an extraordinary mind, which exemplified "the brilliance, the insatiable drive for discovery and the greatest repository of knowledge on the biology of human disease the world has ever known." Dr. Barker believed that low birth weight during the gestational period led to weight gain in later life. He and his team came to this conclusion after poring over data from multigenerational studies of survivors of Hitler's two-and-a-half-year siege of Leningrad (1941–1944), when bread rations for office workers and their dependents dropped to 125 grams—or 250 calories—per day. Called "the fetal origins of adult disease," this theory postulates that there exist specific developmental periods during which an organism is "plastic" or "sensitive" to its environment.[12] In other words, a negative environment *in utero* could lead to the possibility of illness as an adult.

Both Barker's and Widdowson's findings clearly indicate that the environmental factors before and after birth can cause lifelong epigenetic changes: genetic changes that do not involve structural DNA but rather their dysfunction. The mechanism for such epigenetics is a process called methylation of structural genes and, as a result, fetal experiences *before* birth lead to epigenetic changes that persist *after* birth. (The epigenome is the collection of "tags" that can turn genes on or off.) For many of the 30 percent of the global population that carry excess weight, such epigenetic changes become heritable (aka imprinted genes), meaning that they can be passed on to future generations.

Precautions for Expectant Moms with Insulin Resistance

Hundreds of women with insulin resistance who visit our clinic have found it challenging to get pregnant. To aid them in conceiving, our approach is to have them rigorously control their insulin levels with medications if necessary, consume a closely monitored low-carbohydrate diet, and commit to regular exercise. More often than not, this strategy does the trick, enabling them to get pregnant naturally. Next, expectant mothers with insulin resistance should have optimal care *throughout* their pregnancy. Exercise continues to be a key component. By following these recommendations pre-conception and throughout pregnancy, many of the mothers in our clinic community are delighted when they deliver infants of normal weight, which means they have a lower risk for insulin resistance.

The Origin of Our Metabolic Evolution

Recent evidence suggests that groups of our early ancestors may have begun their historic migrations as early as two hundred thousand years ago and interbred with Neanderthals.[13] However, most humans probably migrated out of Africa eighty-five thousand years ago, eventually populating all corners of the world. As a result, *Homo sapiens* shows remarkably little genetic diversity, sharing more than 99 percent of the same DNA. Despite myriad differences in outward appearance, we are all members of one closely evolved superfamily. Approximately thirty thousand years ago, Asian migrants crossed the Bering Strait to Alaska, becoming the first of our species to inhabit the American continent.

One can only imagine the hardships that such people must have endured, especially in finding enough food to survive. The ability to store body fat when food was plentiful enabled our ancestors to later endure periods of food scarcity, an ability centered on insulin resistance. Individuals who possessed those genes had a huge leg up, while those who did not were more likely to perish and therefore not pass along their genes. Insulin resistance was essentially a survival tool, but in the modern world it has become a liability.

The interplay between genes and the environment has been exhaustively studied by examining the differences between Pima Indians living in Arizona and those residing in Mexico. In Pima communities in Arizona, life changed dramatically with the construction of the Coolidge

Dam, completed in 1928, which diverted their water supplies from the Gila River, making farming impossible. By 1965, 46 percent of Pima adults—more women than men—developed type 2 diabetes.[14] With the genetic potential for insulin resistance already in place in this ethnic group (Native Americans, Hispanics, Blacks, South Asians, Africans, and Caribbean Islanders, among others, have higher prevalence rates), the Pima people were dealt a terrible blow to their lifestyle, as well as their well-being. Their metabolic health became severely compromised as they had to rely on government-subsidized, highly processed, trans-fat and corn syrup–infused food. Another Pima group established in an isolated area in Mexico maintained their subsistence farming lifestyle with limited Western influences. In dramatic contrast, here the adult diabetes rate was near 7 percent, less than a fifth of that among their Arizona brethren, although still higher than non-Pimas in the region.[15]

A similar scenario seems to be evolving among the Inuit peoples who migrated from coastal Alaska to Arctic Canada, Greenland, and Siberia a thousand years ago. Their traditional way of life was once dependent upon food sources such as fish, seal, and whale blubber. With the Inuit transition to urban life and a higher consumption of processed, packaged food, excess weight and diabetes continue to rise.[16] As with the Pima, the Inuits from the Bering Strait, from the Nunavik region of Northern Quebec, and others, who have a diabetes prevalence rate averaging 35 percent in the men and women, likely inherited a high prevalence of genes encoded for insulin resistance, an asset for when pickings were slim, but which only became a metabolic liability when their traditional way of life eroded.[17]

Tracking the Mischievous Genetic Messengers

"I was born with a genetic twist in my metabolism, but I think I'm finally winning over it," says Beth, thirty-two, copper-haired, with high cheekbones and the deliberate manner of a person who chooses her words carefully. Her heavyset father and brother, both more than six feet tall, are in and out of doctors' offices as they dodge medical threats on many fronts, including hypertension, coronary heart complications, and elevated liver enzymes. Beth's blood work revealed that she, too, had inherited her father's insulin resistance. At five foot six and 255 pounds, Beth was on the verge of progressing from an Emerald to a Ruby metabolism with a risk for high blood pressure and blood clots in the legs and lungs.

Beth swapped her eighteen-hour-a-day career in Manhattan's digital media world to become a professor at an elite East Coast university. She made this change in order to prioritize her health. She says, "Based on what I witnessed with my father and brother, I saw clearly where my future path would lead me. That I would go from being a well-paid over-achiever to spending my days in hospitals, trying to salvage my health. It took some therapy to disentangle the behavioral aspects—mainly stress—from my professional and family history. For years, I dreaded clothes that didn't fit. But I never dealt with the deep psychological anxiety, which I now realize is part of the insulin resistance spectrum. I've made a lot of progress. But since the underlying causes are genetic, I have to hold myself accountable not to wander off from following diet and health guidelines and have the setbacks I so frequently had during my life in the city."

Clinic Notes

Beth should be proud. Once she understood her dominant genetic legacy, she developed purposeful lifestyle adjustments to restrain her insulin levels. Beth understood that beyond weight loss, the management of insulin resistance necessitates a 360-degree analysis of the effect of genes, stress, sleep, and exercise on metabolic resilience. Over a five-year period, her weight dropped from 255 pounds to 195 pounds. However, in the four years that followed, Beth's inherent genetic tendency asserted itself and she steadily regained the pounds she had lost, accompanied by worsening lipid levels and an enlarged liver. She blamed her setback on her all-consuming work responsibilities, as well as on her meal choices in trendy Manhattan restaurants. Once Beth changed careers, she scheduled regular periods for exercise, relaxation, and sleep and closely followed the MetaKura meal plan for an Emerald metabolism. She decided to stick to the same meal plan every week and take the guesswork out of her diet. It worked. Beth has stopped her medication for anxiety. She tells us that at family gatherings, some relatives don't recognize her. For the last three years, she has maintained her weight at 194 pounds. Witnessing her father's and brother's growing medical complications, Beth rightly believes that she has changed her genetic destiny.

Today 42 percent of American adults are clinically overweight to the degree that it will likely curtail their life span. Despite billions of dollars expended on studies seeking to identify the genes responsible for being overweight, such speculative efforts, like Marcel Proust's (appropriately named) *In Search of Lost Time*, could fill six volumes. While researchers failed to come up with convincing population-wide genetic tests, we *do* know that insulin resistance is heritable.

As if to emphasize the difficulty of this undertaking, only 10 percent of children with severe weight impairment, such as Ariana's Prader-Willi, have rare chromosomal abnormalities.[18] In these rare instances, the identifiable genes with alphabet soup names like MCR4 and POMC all affect the appetite. They have not been shown to be pertinent to the families that we and others see on a daily basis in our clinics who have insulin resistance. Prader-Willi and other rare disorders do, however, show that gene mutations can lead to unwanted body fat.

Twins and the Gemini Study

Sunita is a fraternal twin, born eight minutes before her brother, so we are especially drawn to twin studies. Unlike Sunita and her brother, identical twins start life as a single egg fertilized by a single sperm, which creates a zygote that then splits in two, becoming two embryos with identical genetic makeup. Such monozygotic twins have long been a subject of fascination and research in the efforts to distinguish between genetic and environmental influences on health. A 1986 study of twins by Dr. Albert "Mickey" Stunkard, a pioneer in weight-related research, published in the *New England Journal of Medicine (NEJM)* rocked the world of metabolic medicine.[19,20]

A debonair, silver-haired practicing Buddhist and psychiatrist at the University of Pennsylvania, Stunkard was also the first person to identify binge eating. The groundbreaking *NEJM* study was based on his examination of archived records dating between 1924 and 1946 on 540 adopted Danish twins. He found that among identical twins who had been separated at birth, 70 percent of the male pairs weighed within five to ten pounds of each other as adults. Likewise, 66 percent of the adult female pairs of identical twins weighed about the same, regardless of stark differences in their childhood homes. In a follow-up interview, Stunkard cited an unpublished study of adopted children in Iowa that reached a similar conclusion: contrary to the public's lament about overweight people lacking discipline, environment and lifestyle choices played a mere 30 percent role in determining a person's body weight.[21]

Stunkard's next phase of discovery, published in 1990, upheld this claim. Again, whether raised together or apart, each identical twin's body mass index was nearly the same. The strongest heritability, he said, was found between mothers and biological daughters, followed by mothers and sons.[22] Stunkard's associate, Jane Wardle, PhD, played a leading role in the Gemini Twin Research Study.[23] Gemini Study photographs show a lineup of loose-limbed teenage fraternal twins who share the same DNA as regular siblings. Their similarities are obvious, but the differences in weight, height, and occasionally in coloring are more vivid. The lineup of identical twins is quite another matter.

Dr. Wardle provided further evidence for heritability of weight with her 2008 Twins Early Development Study (TEDS). Annual surveys begun in 1994 confirmed the heritability for both BMI and waist circumference exhibited in identical twins. The study showed that genetics strongly influences the satiety signals that the brain sends to the body when it determines that the body has had enough to eat.[24]

NOAM CHANGES HIS WAYS

 At age forty-three, Noam was further along in his odyssey of metabolism-related complications than Beth because he had been diagnosed with type 2 diabetes. Like the multistrand necklaces that he sells in Manhattan's Diamond District, Noam's family roots are entwined, encompassing Iran, Britain, Israel, India, and now the United States. Both his parents trace their ancestry to Jewish communities that settled in Mashhad, an Iranian city, 2,700 years ago, long before the arrival of Islam. In the 1930s, Noam's father's family moved to England. His mother's parents were part of the diaspora that migrated to India before later settling in Israel. A jovial, swarthy man with deep family attachments, Noam travels across five continents to design, craft, and sell his jewelry.

One of his earliest questions to us was "Why is there so much diabetes on my mother's side of the family?" His mother, as well as her four brothers and two sisters, had all been diagnosed with the condition. "And why do none of my father's relatives have this ailment? Both sides of my family eat exactly the same type of food and have similar ways of life."

As we worked with Noam, we began to probe more deeply into his childhood and life patterns. "My mother cooked like no one else," Noam said. "Every weekend we had Persian-influenced feasts such as *ghormeh sabzi* (lamb braised with spinach and dried lime) with basmati rice. Or *noon toof tone* (cardamom and rose water–flavored meringues). I lived for those moments." Then he added, "I got my bar mitzvah suit in the husky boys' section of the store. All my siblings were chubby."

In addition to the diabetes on his mother's side of the family, Noam acknowledged that "The second factor that weighs against me is that I'm a workaholic." Noam's twelve-hour workday is elongated by incessant travel and a commute from Westchester County into New York City. At his initial assessment, Noam said that his meals tended to revolve around his schedule—he ate meals at home, in the car, and at work. He also told us that he enjoys late family dinners, does not always sleep well, and confesses that every now and then he finds himself very stressed by the quirky world of commerce.

Like many people with an impaired metabolism, Noam's predicament was not for lack of trying to counter the influence of genetics. "I remember sitting on a couch at my heaviest weight of 266 pounds, when I was in my thirties, and I couldn't breathe because my stomach was in the way. Five years after my initial diabetes diagnosis, at the age of forty, I was only losing a couple of pounds per year. My blood sugar was racing upward, on one occasion, increasing in just six weeks. Newly determined, I began to watch my food intake. At first, I would lose weight all week long, only to gain it back by indulging in heavy meals over the weekend or at the Jewish holidays. I did try weight-loss diuretic pills but wasn't impressed with the results."

When Noam came to MetaKura for help, he wanted to reduce his risk of eventually having to take insulin, as his brother does. "Ever present in my mind is the image of my brother Emmanuel giving himself insulin shots. He has faded a bit since my mother passed away, and he doesn't take care of himself. My other brother, Benjamin, is bipolar, and I know now that there is a connection between metabolic and mental health. After talking to you at the clinic, it became clear that if I continued on the same path, instead of taking ten pills a day, I would likely be injecting myself with insulin in ten years. I am here because I want to avoid this scenario at all costs."

Noam's MetaKura Plan

First, we advised Noam to eat every three hours to keep his blood sugar levels steady. "Taking into consideration my crazy work schedule and kosher restrictions, the MetaKura dietitian studied the restaurant menu near my place of work and told me what to order. I was to eat breakfast at seven a.m. and have a protein bar at eleven a.m. Lunch became a salad instead of cheese sandwiches. I was instructed to have another snack at four p.m. before dinner." Following this protocol, Noam steadily dropped eighteen pounds and his average blood sugars (HbA1c levels) improved from 8.5 percent to 5.9 percent. He was also given a fitness routine that combined resistance and aerobic exercise.

Four months later, Noam hit a snag and regained six pounds. The problem was that by the time he arrived home at eight p.m., he was ravenous. "I would clamor to eat within fifteen seconds of my arrival," he said. We suggested that he snack on a green apple and almonds on the way home. Although Noam was resistant to exercise, we urged him to walk more. After six months, he had lost thirty-two pounds.

With his own diabetes and weight now under control, Noam is concerned for his children. "My youngest son was a bit chubby in his early teens. One day, he saw me take ten pills for my diabetes. I think at that moment he decided that he was going to do everything possible to avoid my fate. He told his mother to stop serving rice, flour, and sugar family meals. Now he's extremely lean." At Noam's urging, his newly married daughter, Esther, now follows the MetaKura diet (see Part III).

Noam says, "Now, if I stray from my food regimen, I can feel the effects and I have to sit on a couch and take a nap. So I try to be aware of what I put in my mouth. When I travel overseas with colleagues, they say, 'Noam, go have your protein bar—it's eleven o'clock.' If I don't, I start slowing down mentally and acting like a robot. Finally, I would say that because we as a family have changed our diet and way of living, my children have elected to avoid diabetes. I believe that I have reduced my chance of ever needing insulin injections. I hope that I am right."

Considering that Noam was regular with his medications, this case shows how ineffective medications and conventional medical management can be without a deep analysis of other causal factors, including diet, sleep, stress patterns, and exercise. Noam's case also shows the seemingly dominant mode of metabolic inheritance from his mother's family. All of those family members with type 2 diabetes were, of course, insulin resistant, which can also be seen manifesting in his children who have tested positive for insulin resistance, and one of whom also joined the MetaKura program.

WHAT THE FUTURE HOLDS

Our ability to survive cycles of feast and famine was first described by geneticist James V. Neel as the "thrifty gene" hypothesis.[25] He argued it was the very genetic adaptations enabling the enhanced ability to store body fat from food, especially from carbohydrates, that have led to our current epidemic of overweight and diabetes, leading, in some cases, to a shorter life span projected for our children.

A recent article in the *Journal of Inborn Errors of Metabolism*, inspired by the work of Sir Archibald Garrod, a pioneer in the field and a renowned British physician, describes more than one thousand metabolism-related genetic disorders caused by defects in enzymes, proteins, hormones, and cell receptors.[26] Garrod famously said, "Science is…a way of searching out by observation, trial and classification; whether the phenomena investigated be the outcome of human activities, or of the more direct workings of nature's laws. Its methods admit of nothing untidy or slip-shod; its keynote is accuracy and its goal is truth."

Deciphering all the genetic causes of metabolic imbalances remains a formidable task. Using precision nutrition, a form of personalized nutrition that relies on combining several types of data, genetic, behavioral, and dietary preferences, we and others are now studying the basis for measuring individual and community variances in metabolic response to commonplace nutritional choices.

In the next chapter, you'll learn our rationale for the kinds of foods we advise you to eat and which ones to avoid, choices that have helped thousands of individuals overcome metabolic problems and transform their lives.

CHAPTER 4

Nutritional Profiles: Food, Culture, and Identity

Taste is one of our senses which gives us the greatest joy...
because it can mingle with all other pleasures, and even console
us for their absence.

—Jean Anthelme Brillat-Savarin

Food in all its dazzling and delectable forms is a leading actor, if occasionally one shrouded in mystery, in each of the client stories we hear in our clinic. Nutrition, without doubt, is one of the primary environmental determinants of health. If, as we both believe, human life is a journey of continuous self-discovery, reinvention, and self-acceptance, the twists and turns on this jumbled path are well reflected in the ever-changing relationship with food.

On most weekends, the two of us can be found driving in an elderly silver Prius to scour the farmers' markets in upstate New York for locally sourced heirloom tomatoes, or at seasonal berry farms in the Hudson Valley on the lookout for whole foods of as many varieties as possible. We cook these gems minimally so that they are still rich in nutrients. Food nourishes most when it is seasonal and fresh, so that its connections to the earth and to nature are preserved. We believe that nutritional advice based on biological outcomes offers but a single-dimensional view of food. Instead, we remind ourselves of the deeper meaning of food-sharing rituals, ideas that sustain a cuisine, a culture, and a community. A cuisine, it has been rightly said, is a mirror to the soul of a nation. In his 1921 *Ethnology of the Kwakiutl*, Franz Boas, a towering figure in creating more inclusive precepts in anthropology, recorded that the dining rituals of British Columbia's Coastal First People dictated that water was consumed after an elderberry feast but never after a gooseberry feast.[1] Guests sang special feast songs when they ate rice root. These small gestures conferred a distinct personality on each of these bounties of nature. While honoring these types of culinary philosophies as you imbibe nutrients, your meals sustain you at a deeper level.

Across the ages, in all human societies, preparation of food is a sublime feat of sourcing, creative seasoning, and taste. Richard Wrangham, the primatologist and anthropologist, describes humans as cookivores. "We do not eat cooked food because we have the right kind of teeth and guts; rather we have small teeth and short guts as a result of adapting to a cooked diet."[2] Even if you do not think of yourself as a cookivore, the recipes created by our dear friend Vivian Cioffi (see Chapter 15) are so simple, quick, and delicious that we hope that you will not be able to resist the opportunity to try them out.

The chapters that follow provide a detailed portrait of the foods that we favor for each element of the Metabolic Matrix. Here are a few introductory observations.

SCENES FROM THE METAKURA FOOD LAB

Featured throughout this chapter are vignettes about the foods that are staples in our home and those of our patients. Here, we look at foods for their nutritional properties as well as their distinctive personalities.

Every second, your metabolism busily traffics thousands of enzyme reactions within each cell of your body. These depend on your food choices, so forget counting calories. Instead, as we will show, focus on the foods that will help you better manage the enzyme activity. (See Part III.)

Viva Vegans

 "Even as I was eating one thing, I would be thinking, when am I going to eat next?" said Christina, a cheerful forty-five-year-old with a Ruby metabolism. "My husband would say that I could not possibly be starving one hour after a big meal, but the truth is that I would be craving food. This uncontrollable urge took over my life." Christina is a vegan and, like many, was overly relying on grains in her diet, which led to her unmanageable hunger patterns.

A well-balanced plant-based diet can help people flourish at all stages of life. Drawn from a wide diversity of legumes, grains, vegetables, fruits, nuts, seeds, herbs, and spices, plant-based diets can also meet the needs of pregnant and lactating mothers—with a few caveats. We commonly advise vitamin B_{12} supplementation for vegans, as well as vitamin D_3 if you do not get enough sunlight.

Rather than substituting rice and other starches for animal proteins, go for vegetables instead.

- The legume family is full of protein-rich options. Think soybeans (including edamame), hummus (made with chickpeas), fava beans, kidney beans, lima beans, and so on.
- Sprout mung beans and alfalfa seeds, chia, and sunflower seeds.
- Enjoy pasta made only from red lentils, mung beans, edamame, and other legumes. Be sure to avoid any that are made with added ingredients like tapioca flour or wheat flour.
- Quinoa is an acceptable grain for vegans. It contains all the nine essential amino acids—rare for a plant—that are essential for tissue repair and nutrient absorption, which vegans may not find elsewhere.*

---

* There are nine essential amino acids, which you must get through your diet: histidine, isoleucine, leucine, lysine, methionine, phenylalanine, threonine, tryptophan, and valine.

- If you are unable to cook, pick up a fresh chopped salad, add beans or lentils, and top it with nutritional yeast instead of Parmesan or other cheese.
- Tofu and tempeh are fine protein sources, but avoid seitan and other soy-based foods that contain wheat.
- Nuts, seeds, and their butters are encouraged.
- Become a scrupulous reader of food labels to avoid sugar, sugar alcohols, corn syrup, agave, and molasses, as well as any additives.

Healing Vegetables and Fruits

The more that you prepare your own food, however simply, the greater control you have over the ingredients interacting with your metabolism.

Cabbage, an Ancient Cultivar: Despite being one of the oldest cultivated vegetables, cabbage doesn't get the respect it merits. This cruciferous vegetable, of which there are four hundred varieties—valued by the odd bedfellows Pliny and Captain Cook for its healing properties—is rich in antioxidants and fiber. Fermented as sauerkraut and kimchi, it's a recommended prebiotic food. Among the zesty cabbage recipes we enjoy is one infused with turmeric, toasted mustard seeds, and a hint of chili pepper.

The Fruits of Labor: Watermelons, mangoes, kiwis, and others are ill-advised for regular consumption, as, being high in fructose, they increase the glycemic load on the metabolism. High sugar content increases food cravings and, more worryingly, has been implicated in an increased risk for depression and other mental illness.[3] Instead, we favor Granny Smith apples. These apples, the story goes, originated in 1868 in New South Wales, Australia, when Maria Ann Smith tossed away the remains of Tasmanian crab apples. In one popular study, the fruit pulp of organic Granny Smith apples showed the highest microbial diversity compared to other apple varietals.[4] Note that baked apples have an increased sugar content, as cooking liberates sweet-tasting fructose.

We champion berries of every variety. Strawberries are a symbol of blessing among the Iroquois and had sacred medicinal qualities for the

Navajo people. Strawberries are rich in both fisetin and quercetin, which belong to a family of micronutrients called plant flavonoids and are associated with anti-aging and reducing inflammation and the risk for coronary disease. Blueberries, rich in antioxidants, fiber, and vitamin C, were also used by the earliest Native Americans as natural medicines.

Hunger-Stimulating Foods

 For Colin and many people like him, their choice of food is determined by the degree of comfort that it offers in what they perceive to be a merciless world. Unfortunately, many of these choices actually induce hunger. Colin joined the MetaKura program to address his sleep apnea, episodic high blood pressure, and abnormal lipid profile. He was also forty pounds above his ideal body weight.

"Doc," he said, "look at my life. These days you get calls and emails twenty-four-seven. When my phone rings at ten p.m. and there's a trader calling from London, I can't complain because it's four a.m. there." Colin is forty-two and a partner in a private equity firm. "When Wall Street guys have a few minutes to relax, they turn to cigar bars, steak dinners, and other stuff. There's a sense that you've *earned* these rare moments of pleasure for all the hours of stress you've put yourself through, and then before you know it, you are addicted to an expensive habit."

Colin said, "As I've been piecing it together, my Greek family's high-calorie diet from their farming days never changed. Sharing food was critical to strengthening family bonds. The dinner table was where we talked. For my mother and perhaps for the rest of us too, food was a consolation for any disappointments in life."

Colin's current eating style did not involve sitting at the family table. He said, "We order in at work a lot. It's probably not the healthiest diet." He returned to the connection between his newly diagnosed health complications and his work-related stress. "Look at the way my compensation is structured. If you get a package of, for argument's sake, $1 million, then $200,000 is your salary. The remaining $800,000 is held back as your bonus. Everything you do all year round, you keep in mind that after New Year's Day, only if all goes well with you and your firm's performance, you will get your due." He also confessed to some difficulty concentrating. "If someone embarks on a very complicated discussion, after thirty minutes or so, I will likely have lost the thread."

Colin told us that he felt tired when he woke up in the morning. Colin dropped his head as he lowered his voice. "To tell you the truth, these days I feel down more often. I keep telling myself that I have the perfect life, a great career, a beautiful wife, home, and family. I want to be healthy for them."

Clinic Notes

At five feet eleven inches tall and 269 pounds, Colin had a long history of yo-yo weight cycles, high triglyceride levels, and intermittent elevated blood pressure. He had been born at full term with a smaller than average birth weight of six pounds seven ounces. Colin had multiple skin tags and dark shadows (*acanthosis nigricans*) on his neck. His underlying insulin resistance was confirmed by laboratory testing. Colin's mother had been diagnosed with type 2 diabetes. His father was slim but had suffered two heart attacks and had high blood pressure. Colin often worked late, and his office food choices were not optimal. We encouraged him to make time for breakfast. Numerous studies* have concluded that "eating breakfast was associated with significantly lower coronary heart disease risk."[5]

People such as Colin typically have elevated levels of triglycerides—his were 365 mg/dL, while a normal level is less than 140 mg/dL. When such people eat simple carbohydrate foods, despite their insulin level being twice or four times the norm, the insulin fails to prevent fat cells from releasing fatty acids. This results in the high triglyceride levels and persistently low levels of high-density lipoproteins (HDL) often seen in the blood of insulin-resistant people.

---

* A 2013 study funded by the NIH and published by L. E. Cahill et al., they reported on data from 51,529 healthy males (monitored from 1992 up to 2008).

High insulin levels also impair the kidneys' ability to excrete salt. As salt is retained, blood volume increases, which in turn raises blood pressure. Colin required medication to bring his elevated blood pressure of 156/92 down to normal. In this case, his elevated blood pressure mirrored his levels of stress. As Colin lowered his insulin responses by making changes in his diet, his blood pressure settled into a consistently normal range, as did his uric acid level (5.4 mg/dL).

Colin was able to reverse his medical complications primarily with minor changes to his meals. At our three-month review, Colin had mostly adhered to his diet plan. In the morning, he ate eggs or Greek yogurt with berries. We advised him to try to limit the yogurt to one two-ounce container at one time, because while yogurt is a complex carbohydrate, it is an energy-dense food. For lunch, he ate either salmon, chicken, or a burger without bread. His biggest obstacle was trying to avoid fried or breaded appetizers while entertaining large groups of clients. By having a snack of nuts or green apples with cheese before going out for dinner, Colin was able to decrease his hunger level. We offered Colin several options when he craved bread or pasta.

Instead of sacrificing your favorite foods, prepare them with creative substitutes.

Alternatives for Bread and Pasta

- Almond flour muffins
- Spelt flour or sprouted Ezekiel bread
- Buckwheat soba noodles
- Indian buckwheat flour (*kuttu ka atta*)
- Black bean pasta, lentil pasta, chickpea pasta (Make sure such products contain 100 percent of the permitted ingredient with no added flours.)

Buckwheat: A Nutritious Imposter

If it looks like a duck and quacks like a duck, don't assume anything. Such is the case of buckwheat. It may appear to be a grain, but it is actually related to the vegetable rhubarb and the herb sorrel. Believed to have been cultivated in China as early as 4000 BCE, buckwheat contains all of the nine amino acids that humans cannot produce. It also has a high fiber content of 4.5 grams per cup. Both these factors make it popular globally—in the form of soba noodles in Japan, kasha porridge in Eastern Europe, galette crepes in Brittany, France, and *kuttu ka atta,* an Indian flatbread associated with the Navaratri festival. Buckwheat was brought to Russia by invading Tartars in the sixteenth century, and kasha (a porridge) imagery suffuses the Russian language. "He has kasha in his head" (instead of brains) or "to cook kasha with someone" (to talk turkey with someone) are popular expressions.

Brain Boosters

For many years, Marilyn, a fifty-three-year-old senior financial director at a government agency, accompanied her twenty-eight-year-old daughter, Theresa, to our clinic. Theresa has type 1 diabetes, which she manages superbly by meticulously following every instruction provided to her. Marilyn's life has not been easy. Born in Kaohsiung, Taiwan, she arrived in Brooklyn as an eleven-year-old to join her parents, who worked in a sportswear factory in Manhattan's Chinatown. She spoke no English. Marilyn said that she overcame the initial years of racist schoolyard bullying thanks to her proficiency in martial arts. Soon she was president of her class in high school and later earned a full college scholarship and went on to graduate with a degree in computer science. Twenty years ago, after her husband left the family, Marilyn found herself as a single mother supporting three children, including Theresa. Extremely hardworking, Marilyn excelled at her career with a series of technology companies, including those that provided outsourced services to a government agency; she is now currently employed at that agency.

"I was used to a work culture that was busier, where there was more accountability. My new boss didn't have my back and I got my first-ever average performance appraisal at work," Marilyn said when she joined the MetaKura program. "It caused a huge emotional upheaval for me.

For months, I've stopped exercising and I haven't got enough sleep. I've been eating anything in sight, cookies, bread, or pasta. I've gained forty pounds. I was constantly tired, sad, had difficulty concentrating, and found that I had short-term memory loss. But as soon as I found out that Theresa was pregnant, I knew that I had to get my act together so that I could be there for my daughter with diabetes and for my grandchild."

As she has always done, six months later, Marilyn delivered on her promise. The MetaKura program resolved Marilyn's hypertension. She attributed her thirty-eight-pound weight loss to eating more selectively, adding salmon and other omega fatty acids to her diet, and to weighing herself every morning. Marilyn said her concentration has improved and she feels more optimistic. She invested in an exercise bike, lifts weights when she watches TV, and sleeps more than she did previously. Marilyn joyfully announced on her last visit that her eldest daughter is about to deliver her second grandchild.

Mood Food

A common side effect of insulin resistance is "brain fogginess," short-term memory loss, or difficulty with concentration, especially after eating sugary foods that elevate insulin levels. Especially helpful for brain health are the following:

- Omega fatty acids[6] (found in salmon, walnuts, flax, and chia seeds) have been used to treat mood disorders.
- Vitamin D (found in soy milk, mushrooms, and cheese) and vitamin E (found in avocado, peanuts, and olives) improve brain health after middle age.
- Iron (found in lentils, beans, and poultry) has been shown to be beneficial in restoring cognitive function in highly anemic young women of reproductive age.[7]
- Choline (found in bok choy, cabbage, and eggs) has been seen to modulate neuroplasticity, although the data is mixed.

Smooth Operator

"Doctor, can you solve a mystery? I watch my calories, run in the park every day, and yet I'm gaining weight," said thirty-six-year-old Luisa at her first clinic appointment.

Among the changes we suggested was that Luisa forgo her daily green smoothies.

Even if one succeeds in avoiding a smoothie's hidden sugars (according to dietitian Marlene Koch, an average smoothie can contain a half cup of sugar),[8] research shows that consuming liquids is less efficient than eating solid food at enabling you to feel satisfied with your meal.[9] The American food faddist Horace Fletcher (1849–1919) put forth the doctrine "nature will castigate those who don't masticate," an admonition that has stood the test of time. Studies by Hélène Labouré and others reveal that consuming a soup purée resulted in increased triglyceride and insulin responses when compared to eating the same ingredients minimally cooked and whole.[10]

Also beware the cleansing trend that has become the equivalent of a spiritual retreat. The liver and kidneys are well designed to remove toxins from the body. A purging cleanse may very transiently induce weight loss due to water depletion but can deprive your body of essential nutrients. Instead of purging, we suggest indulging in a cocoa drink.

Cacao Beans: Food of the Gods

Archaeological finds of Mayan vases reveal a sophisticated culture of imbibing foamy cacao. In the 1570s, a Renaissance botanist, Francisco Hernández, royal physician to Philip II of Spain, created a folio of drawings that recorded Aztec reverence for *cacahua cuahuitl* (the cacao tree).[11] The plant was named *Theobroma cacao* by the Swedish naturalist Carl Linnaeus (1707–1778). In the 1600s, the Venezuelan cities of Maracaibo and Caracas became leading centers for exporting the finest cacao. A drink of water-based cocoa (75 percent cacao) is truly a divine gift to your body, rich in antioxidants, fiber, and anti-inflammatory properties.

Eye-Watering Tales and Salty Stories

 James, a bearded, fast-talking sixty-five-year-old owner of a talent agency, had noticeable facial twitches and compulsions like constantly checking his phone. He came to the clinic soon after being discharged from a Manhattan hospital with a muddled diagnosis indicating a possible stroke. The problem was that exhaustive imaging studies failed to show evidence of brain hemorrhage or thrombosis. Puzzled, we tried to make sense of the clues. An incidental finding in his blood work was a low serum sodium level, which resulted in modestly elevated blood pressure. Then we noticed that tucked under his chair was James's outsized bottle of water. Excessive consumption of water in older patients is recognized to cause hypertension. When asked to compile a log of all the fluids he consumed throughout the day, including beverages and other drinks, it was two and a half to three times the normal amount. On one hand, switching to a low-carbohydrate diet increases a person's hydration needs for regular gut health. On the other, we see drinking water to excess to be harmful, if not dangerous. The daily fluid requirement for a 150-pound man is about ten cups, including the water found in the food and beverages he consumes. An average-size woman requires about eight cups. James tried to gradually restrict fluid intake by 5 percent a week and was temporarily successful at normalizing his sodium level, but then he reverted to his previous pattern. He drank water compulsively until he started to feel faint, after which he cut back again.

The four common misconceptions that cause people to drink excessive quantities of water include improving one's complexion, weight loss, lowering blood glucose levels (for people with diabetes), and eliminating body toxins. If water and other fluid intake doubles or trebles, a person can develop "water toxicity." This induces the kidneys to produce large amounts of dilute urine, which lowers levels of sodium and chloride in the blood. If these levels become very low, headaches, nausea, mental confusion, faintness, seizures, or even a coma may occur. As blood becomes diluted, water can enter the brain, causing neurons to swell. A gradual reduction in intake starts with keeping a fluid log for several days, followed by a reduction of 5 to 10 percent a week until a doctor advises you that your sodium levels have risen to normal.

We also frequently see examples of ill-advised salt restriction (the US government's dietary guidelines recommend 2,300 mg of sodium per day), which leads to dehydration, low blood pressure, and fainting. This is more likely to occur when a person is in a crowded space or during hot, humid weather. Traveling from a temperate climate such as Seattle to a tropical one such as Antigua, the adrenal gland adapts to this shift by secreting the salt-retaining hormone aldosterone. This process may take about three weeks, during which the individual is most vulnerable to salt depletion.

TWO INSTANT MESSAGING SYSTEMS

A friend's late father, who was an ambassador to Austria from an Asian nation, would return home after a two-hour state banquet at the Hofburg Palace in Vienna, where seven to ten courses of rich cuisine were served. Before going to bed, he would still need to have a bowl of rice.

Biology and culture are said to be the two great rivers of human continuity and change. Our biology is a complex messaging system so powerful that its telltale imprint can be traced in every cell and organ of the body. Culture defines who we are and becomes our internal voice, which fundamentally influences the innumerable nutritional choices that we make each day. T. S. Eliot suggested, "If we take culture seriously, we see that a people does not need merely enough to eat but a proper and particular cuisine; culture may even be described simply as that which makes life worth living."[12]

Rice: A Sacred Though Harmful Grain

The etymology of Buddha's father Suddhodana's name is "pure rice." Mizuho-no-kuni, a name for Japan in old Japanese 瑞穂国, means "country of lush grains (of rice)." Toyoda, the inspiration for Toyota, means "fertile rice paddies"; Honda, the original rice field; Tanaka, dweller in a rice paddy, and Narita, the developing rice field.[13] For people with insulin resistance, we recommend substituting riced cauliflower, finely sliced cabbage, or new brands of rice made only with lentils.

Teach Your Children Well

Our childhood memories are indelibly steeped in the scents and flavors of our family meals. Sadly, today the revered grains and ethnic foods that are the mainstay of billions of humans are now shortening children's lives with metabolism-related chronic conditions. We should not allow our children to believe that hyper-processed snacks or sugar-infused cereals or juices can be considered food, regardless of their packaging claims.

Parents can help their children by forming dietary habits that will enable them to avoid metabolic complications. Keep your kitchen pantry well stocked with nuts and nut products like peanut butter and almond flour, seeds, and (preferably homemade) chickpea flour snacks instead of relying on ultra-processed packaged foods. We recommend ancient grains like spelt flour and buckwheat.

Valerie, a sales-driven real estate agent, jokes that she spent so much time selling homes to others that she barely saw her own. Like many New Yorkers, she does not cook, preferring to eat out or order in. Suffice it to say, the more you do so, the less control you have over the ingredients in your food.

Alexandre Dumas, in his *Grand Dictionary of Cuisine,* wrote, "It is not enough to eat. To dine, there must be diversified, calm conversation.

It should sparkle with the rubies of the wine between the courses, be deliciously suave with the sweetness of dessert, and acquire true profundity with the coffee."

VITAMINS AND SUPPLEMENTS: EFFECTIVE OR SNAKE OIL?

On Whitney's initial visit to the clinic, she had a swollen face and her hands trembled.

Another physician had diagnosed her with adrenal fatigue (usually a phantom ailment, in our view) and then encouraged her to purchase high doses of his clinic's private-label supplements, which had eventually poisoned her.

The idea that supplements promise good health, regardless of a person's frugal exercise routine or fulsome diet, is so appealing that in the United States alone, they enjoy an annual market of $30 billion. Remarkably, the FDA has no requirement that a supplement prove that it delivers the claimed benefit.* Nor does the underfunded FDA perform analyses on these nutrients. When independent labs have tested for their purity and label accuracy, vitamins and supplements have been shown to include toxic and other harmful contaminants. Or they have a complete absence (or minor traces) of their touted active ingredients. From a physician's perspective, this deficient regulation of supplements, far below that of prescription drugs, is shameful. Faced with a healthcare system that is unacceptably expensive, it is not surprising that more people are turning to do-it-yourself treatments for their ailments complemented by self-administered micronutrients.

When undertaken in concert with eating well and exercising, some supplementation can help to counter deficiencies. Below is a list of supplements that, while not comprehensive, are among the ones most prescribed at our clinic.

---

* A 1994 statute gave oversight to the FDA under Dietary Supplements for the Exercise and Athletic Performance Act.

Common Micronutrient Deficiencies

Many women come to the clinic concerned about hair loss. In addition to high levels of testosterone in insulin-resistant individuals, there are at least three relevant micronutrient deficiencies that cause hair loss.

First, we commonly see zinc deficiency. Taking zinc supplements of twenty-five to fifty milligrams daily can be helpful, initially with reducing hair loss, and over a few months, with increased hair volume. Vegans should also be mindful that phytates, antioxidant compounds found in foods such as rice, grains, and corn, may bind enough zinc to lead to overt zinc deficiency, which can affect growth, immunity, and neurological function.

The next common micronutrient deficit is iron, which may cause anemia. The average adult has one to three grams of iron stored in his or her body.[14] Here again, women need special attention. They lose iron via menstruation, and as many as 50 percent of women with autoimmune thyroid disease have a related complication that results in iron deficiencies. Atrophic gastritis is an autoimmune condition of the stomach lining in which acid secretion declines, and this leads to a progressive decline in the absorption of iron. In later life, vitamin B_{12} absorption also becomes impaired.

Thirdly, we see a deficiency of amino acids, the building blocks for protein, especially sulphur-containing cysteine and homocysteine. Increasing intake of animal protein such as eggs and cheese will help alleviate this problem, but for dedicated vegans, quinoa has more essential amino acids than most grains. Without proteins, there would be no insulin and no life. Omega fatty acid supplements have long been endorsed to facilitate heart health, but positive evidence that they were effective was lacking and their efficacy was recently refuted.[15]

Deficiencies of vitamins, especially the fat-soluble ones of A, D, E, and K, and minerals can also occur in autoimmune intestinal diseases such as celiac disease, ulcerative colitis, and Crohn's disease.

Take Supplements with Care

We do not cover all supplements comprehensively, only the ones that we commonly suggest to our patients. Per FDA rules, physicians can only prescribe vitamin D_2 (which is less beneficial than D_3) and only in the amount of fifty thousand units, which can cause toxicity. We've had rafts of patients poisoned by too much vitamin D, which places them at risk for kidney stones and neurological damage caused by abnormally elevated calcium levels.

Speaking of calcium, we do not prescribe it as supplement. There is no evidence that calcium supplements improve or prevent osteoporosis. Such supplements have been shown to be associated with an increased rate of Alzheimer's, at least in women.

Sift through the most compelling factors that determine your food choices, from availability, habit, social, cultural, and financial considerations. Then resolve that if you are a Sapphire, Emerald, or Ruby metabolism, the most crucial choice for you is the extent to which your dietary choices will restore order to your metabolic imbalances. Always keep in mind the biochemical benefits of "commensality," or sharing meals with others. Julia Child said, "You don't have to cook fancy or complicated masterpieces—just good food from fresh ingredients."

CHAPTER 5

Hunger: Signals That Fine-Tune the Appetite

I can reason down or deny everything, except this perpetual
Belly: feed he must and will, and I cannot make him respectable.
—Ralph Waldo Emerson, American essayist and
poet (1803–1882)

With a cavelike mouth oozing venom and a camouflage of yellow, orange, and black skin, Gila monsters can store eight weeks of survival sustenance in their torpedo-shaped tails. In 1990, this feat of gastroplasticity caught the attention of Harvard-educated Dr. John Eng, who worked at the Veterans Administration (VA) hospital in the Bronx, New York. He also did research at the labs of Rosalyn Yalow, who had devised a new way to measure hormones such as insulin, using radioisotopes. Dr. Eng and his colleagues announced that after years of experimental studies on nature-made hunger modulating enzymes in chinchillas and guinea pigs, they had identified a new hormone in the Gila monster's venom. Their new discovery, named exendin-4, is what enabled the lizard to slow down its metabolism, control its appetite, and maintain steady blood sugar levels during long periods of fasting, without any ill effects.

Thrillingly to Eng, exendin-4, which he described as "his fifth child," was 52 percent identical in structure and function to a human hormone, glucagon-like peptide-1 (GLP-1), found in the lower intestine, which also suppresses appetite and stimulates pancreatic insulin production. There was one important difference. GLP-1 action in the body is abruptly curtailed by an enzyme named dipeptidyl peptidase-4 (DPP-4), which accounts for its short biological life, whereas lab-made exendin-4 can resist this action. After food is eaten, GLP-1 is active in the human body for about two minutes, while exendin-4, by dodging the control of domineering enzymes, can remain functional for several hours, suggesting that it could be an effective treatment for controlling appetite and diabetes.*

The VA declined to patent Eng's discovery of exendin-4 because it did not address a veteran-specific ailment, such as spinal cord damage or another combat injury, so he decided to patent it himself.[1] He prevailed, received the patent, and the know-how for regulating insulin levels was later acquired by a pharmaceutical company for $325 million in September 2002.[2] Since then, it has led to at least six GLP-1 and DPP-4–related therapies for managing diabetes, satiety, and hunger. Due to its glycemic control capabilities, these drugs are also being studied as treatments for Alzheimer's.[3]

HUNGER OR APPETITE: WHO'S IN CHARGE?

In his *Journal of the Private Life and Conversations of the Emperor Napoleon at St. Helena*, Emmanuel, Count of Las Cases, quoted the French statesman and military leader as saying, "Such is the influence of the belly. It is hunger that rules the world." Biologically, hunger is an urgent nutritional need that, if ignored, can induce a feeling of light-headedness. Resisting this sensation, as many do for religious purposes, is seen as ennobling. In addition to being motivated to lose weight, intermittant fasters may feel a sense of moral superiority at having conquered this most basic of human instincts. In Ernest Hemingway's *A Moveable Feast,*

---

* A problem with GLP-1 analogues is that they are hormones and have to be injected. However, inhibitors of the DDP-4 enzyme have been developed that have GLP-1 actions and can be given orally as a tablet. Since weight reduction from GLP-1 agonists is modest, the authors have a strong bias to the DPP-4s in the treatment of diabetes.

set in 1920s Paris, hunger changes the cash-poor writer's experience at the Luxembourg Museum: "...all the paintings were sharpened and clearer and more beautiful if you were belly-empty and hollow-hungry."[4] Conversely, the notion of appetite is still steeped in religious admonishments and the psychology of self-indulgence.

Say Nay to Plus Ultra

At a time when 70 percent of the calories we consume come from processed food (some of which is minimally processed and on our recommended list like peanut butter, Greek yogurt, or hummus), leading global voices like Carlos Monteiro, professor of nutrition at the University of São Paulo, are raising the alarm. Ultra-processed foods, he says, which include breakfast cereals, ice cream, crackers, and cookies, are typically manufactured with highly flavorful ingredients and have engaging marketing campaigns to promote them. Over time, as their sugar and fat flavors become associated with satiety cues, they override the body's built-in mechanisms for appetite regulation.[5]

According to Monteiro, these products are no longer foods but perversions of technology: "You take some high yield crops, and you use them in a way to extract the cheapest protein, the cheapest oil, the cheap carb. And then you recombine them into a product of very low cost. The formulation of these products actually aims to fool our bodies to consume more than we need. So in a way, we lose the ability to control the amount of food we need because we are not really consuming food. We are consuming these hyper-palatable formulations."

Monteiro adds that food manufacturers are adding dozens of new additives that increase our cravings for these cheap, nutrition-stripped products.[6] Discourse around food has, over the years, only grown more argumentative. Prompted by long-overdue conversations on the ethics of food consumption, ever-growing types of diets (ours among them), including keto, paleo, high-protein, low-fat, plant-based, and vegan, combined with widespread confusion about the nutritional values of trendy "superfoods," have many people anxious about their food choices.

Arturo Hungers for More

Arturo, fifty-eight, is a psychologist who leads a suicide prevention program in Brooklyn. His elderly parents had been longtime patients of the clinic until the end of their lives. He says, "We Americans as a society have not learned how to tolerate discomfort. People rush to seek solace in food, gambling, or drugs to soothe their sense of unease. Individuals who have an internal locus of control, ones who are okay with managing discomfort, have a lower risk for high anxiety or suicide. The others, who depend on external factors like luck or fate, are more vulnerable."

His earliest childhood memories, Arturo says, included food-centered Sunday meals with his grandparents, where pizza, chicken and potatoes, meatballs, pastrami sandwiches, and Chinese fried rice featured on their standard menu. By thirty-five years of age, after he was married and had two children, Arturo says, his craving for foods like an eggplant parmesan hero or for fried, breaded chicken was like an addiction. "My appetite was utterly out of control," he says. Three years ago, after a painful episode of kidney stones, Arturo adapted to the MetaKura way of life. To his enormous relief, after losing forty pounds, his calf twitches, which were once suspected to be a symptom of a life-threatening neuromotor disease, have disappeared. "I consume half the portions of food that I once did," he says. "Changing my diet has significantly reduced my hunger."

As societies become more alert to the appetite-signaling changes that arise from the habitual consumption of most grains, the next frontier, we believe, is to acknowledge the effects of fructose—sugar absorbed directly into the bloodstream. Perhaps one of the areas of the Meta-Kura program that elicits the most conversation is the narrow range of fruits that we favor. Unlike glucose, which is distributed throughout the body, fructose is metabolized only in the liver and is likelier to cause fat accumulation. When not consumed in moderation, fructose activates neurobiological pathways involved in appetite regulation, thereby promoting increased food responses, especially in the brain's visual cortex and left orbital frontal cortex. In a 2015 study conducted at the University of Southern California that compared the after-effects of drinking seventy-five grams of fructose with an equivalent dose of glucose, a greater appetite and desire for food occured with fructose consumption. Following a fructose drink, subjects were even willing to give up long-term monetary rewards to obtain immediate high-calorie food rewards.[7]

THE MYTH OF A GENERATION

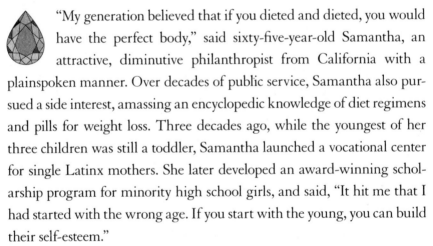 "My generation believed that if you dieted and dieted, you would have the perfect body," said sixty-five-year-old Samantha, an attractive, diminutive philanthropist from California with a plainspoken manner. Over decades of public service, Samantha also pursued a side interest, amassing an encyclopedic knowledge of diet regimens and pills for weight loss. Three decades ago, while the youngest of her three children was still a toddler, Samantha launched a vocational center for single Latinx mothers. She later developed an award-winning scholarship program for minority high school girls, and said, "It hit me that I had started with the wrong age. If you start with the young, you can build their self-esteem."

After serving on a number of educational, regional, and national boards, Samantha recalled the moment that she was elected to serve on the board of one of the country's leading nonprofits for women. She said, "The former president took me aside and said, 'Samantha, you're beautiful, talented, and smart. But you're too fat.' This happened at a time when I was at my heaviest. It was a motivating wake-up call," she said matter-of-factly. "You think people don't see your extra pounds, but they do."

Samantha continued in her upbeat manner: "The most luck in life is getting the right parents. It's not just the DNA, it's people who love and appreciate you. My parents gave me such self-esteem. I never felt insecure. Even though I ended up in a terrible first marriage, no one could take away my sense of purpose—to make a contribution."

At the age of sixteen, Samantha recalled, "I went from 114 to 134 pounds. Mother took me to our family doctor, and that turned out to be a tremendous mistake. He put me on these orange amphetamine diet pills. I lost twenty pounds, but I was jittery and depressed. Years later, I tried everything, including fen-phen diet pills, to slim down. The doctor who prescribed me the drug got arrested because he was also running a meth lab! I lost thirty pounds and then developed a heart issue with the fen-phen. If someone asked me today what I would change about my life, the one thing would be to not have to worry about my weight."

Eight months after Samantha and her husband joined the MetaKura program, she said, "There is no question that sugar and flour make one hungrier. I have noticed that we eat far less now. My increased energy makes me feel younger. I'm more in control than I've ever been."

Clinic Notes

At five feet three inches tall, Samantha weighed 176 pounds. Her paternal grandparent had a notable history of cardiovascular disease. Her father had his first heart attack at age forty-four and lived until he was seventy-nine. Her brother has also had heart surgery. On her mother's side of the family, an aunt had Alzheimer's.

Samantha loved spice-infused cuisines. The first step in making changes was to add a full range of vegetables and selected fruits to her Ruby metabolism diet. This improved her feeling of satiety after meals and, with it, reduced her urge for calorie-dense, late-night snacks. It also made it more likely that she could adhere to her dietary guidelines over the long term.[8]

Samantha's observations about appetite-triggering foods were correct. Complex carbohydrate foods, unlike the simple varieties, are digested more slowly. This delays their absorption and better stimulates GLP-1 secretion from the lower intestine.

A meta-analysis of nine studies found that complex carbs like beans increased satiety by 31 percent.[9] Legumes are also rich in protein, considered the most satiating macronutrient, and which is most beneficial for weight loss and weight maintenance. Beans (legumes) have a dietary fiber content of 5.2 to 7.8 grams per 100 grams, as well as other nutrients such as iron, folate, and calcium.

As for Samantha's fondness for bread, consuming such foods on an empty stomach can induce a rapid release of insulin and a jitter-inducing reactive form of hypoglycemia. This drop in blood sugar creates the urge to eat more food. Repetition of such cycles can lead to recurrent carbohydrate craving.

Thanks to her busy public role, Samantha seldom dined at home, which presented a challenge to her ability to control her appetite. We encouraged her to eat a light snack of nuts or a Granny Smith apple with cheese or peanut butter before attending a social or business event. Our dietitian also studied the menus of restaurants Samantha frequently patronized and guided her meal choices in advance. Two weeks after joining the program Samantha showed limited improvements in her metabolism, so we took a closer look at the ingredients in the foods she was eating. She, more than us, was shocked to find that added sugar lurked in the tuna and egg salads that she ordered at a local deli, rostisserie chicken, and in all nine types of turkey breast sold in her favorite specialty food store. Once she eliminated such foods, her persistent hunger subsided. Samantha has maintained her weight loss of twenty-two pounds.

Appetite and food consumption arises from a complex interplay between biology, psychology, and culture. For others, especially those with insulin dysfunction, these appetite signals are imbalanced. Nuno Casanova and John Blundell of the University of Leeds and other scientists suggest that appetite and food intake are not subject to the same degree of tight biological regulation as other physiological processes such as that of thermoregulation (the maintenance of body temperature).[10]

PLASTICS: OH NO

Jean Anthelme Brillat-Savarin famously said, "Tell me what you eat and I will tell you what you are," but we may also be what our mothers ate. The embryo seems to be especially susceptible to nutrient-induced adaptations in gene expression, a phenomenon referred to as *metabolic imprinting* or *metabolic programming*. In 2003, Randy Jirtle, an American biologist with an expertise in epigenetics, exposed pregnant black mice to an endocrine disrupting chemical called bisphenol A (BPA), commonly found in plastic water bottles and containers worldwide. When the litter was born, a few pups looked starkly different. They had a genetic deviation that caused a tawny golden (agouti) coat quite unlike their black-coated siblings. With this genetic change, there is an overproduction of the AGRP protein that passes to the hypothalamus, blocks satiety signaling, and induces overeating and immense plumpness in the agouti mice. It is thought that a similar blocking action in muscles leads the mice to become insulin resistant. It is also known that bisphenol A is an endocrine disrupter, but other substances increase the prenatal methylation (silences or imprints) of genes as well.

In the next phase of the experiment, Jirtle and his colleagues exposed the pregnant mouse to dietary supplementation like choline, betaine, folic acid, and vitamin B_{12}. This decreased the incidence of agouti mice pups, which was associated with a reduction in their risk of developing obesity, diabetes, and cancer.[11] Could the same effect be occuring in humans?

In discussing decoding appetite regulation, we must pay tribute to biopsychologist John Blundell. He and his colleagues have identified the challenges that humans, as omnivores, face in making optimal food selections. *The omnivore's dilemma* is a phrase coined in 1976 by Paul Rozin, a University of Pennsylvania psychologist, to describe the moral and emotional perils of the human ability to eat anything. This, Blundell says, has made us especially vulnerable to "processed food with strong sensory appeal." He and his colleagues have described hunger as "the result of a cascading dialogue between our outer cultural, social, emotional selves and our internal metabolism-related blueprint."[12] The challenge for people with insulin resistance is that their appetite signals—primarily the satiety hormone leptin, which triggers a feeling of fullness—can get blunted. This, in turn, affects their drive to eat more. Their unsettled appetites may urge them to veer toward the wrong *types* of food and then *also* to struggle with the ability to control the *amount* of food they consume.

CLAIRE'S ASSERTIVE APPETITE SIGNALS

Part of the success of people who have come through our clinic results from a better understanding of the more subtle nuances of their metabolism, especially their underlying appetite deviations. Claire, thirty-six, is a banker with a calm and methodical temperament who said she works in "a shark tank." She told us that one New Year's Eve, after ending a ten-year relationship with the wrong man, she wrote a detailed five-year plan for all the changes she wanted to make in her life. "The first item," she explained, "was to feel better in my body because all your experiences of life—sensory, emotional, intellectual—flow through your physical being."

Claire said, "After six months on the MetaKura program, I've lost twenty-six pounds. I'm very happy to achieve this goal, but I wouldn't say that I'm confident that I can do this forever. I know that part of my problem is that if I eat bread or chocolate, it's hard for me to control my intake." Claire had recently been visiting her father in Paris. "We were invited to a friend's house. I was hungry and the only food being offered were French pralines and Christmas cookies. I probably ate six. But the next day, I stopped myself from any further indulgences."

THE YIN-YANG OF ENERGY NEEDS

"Unquiet meals make ill digestions," the Abbess chides Adriana for being a jealous wife in Shakespeare's *The Comedy of Errors*.[13] Let's stay with this theatrical analogy to explore some of the influences on hunger. When ghrelin, the lead actor and a stomach-hunger (orexigenic) hormone, is injected intravenously, it activates three regions of the brain that direct food intake. These include (1) the midbrain hypothalamus, which links the neurons to hormones in the pituitary gland; (2) the medulla and pons in the brain stem; and (3) the hedonic regions such as the ventral midbrain. Ghrelin then fires up a coterie of supporting-role actors: other hunger-inducing neuropeptides, agouti-related peptide (AGRP) and neuropeptide Y(NPY), which block the appetite-suppressing (anorexigenic) effects of the fat-cell hormone leptin. For our survival, this interplay of interactive neuronal cross talk centered in the hypothalamus is naturally biased to hunger signaling, to ensure that there is sufficient nutrient intake for the body's energy needs. Indeed, as we know, to ensure our survival in periods of feast and famine, there is greater evolutionary tolerance for over-nutrition than for under-nutrition.

Hardwired to pursue food and sex, our midbrain dopamine receptors enable us to predict reward.[14] We know that defective insulin signaling is associated with fatigue, depression, and even bipolar disorders. Brain imaging studies have shown compelling evidence of increased activity of the neurotransmitter dopamine in reinforcing the effects of drug abuse in humans in the striatum area of the brain.[15] Cellular physiologist Lynette Daws and her colleagues have researched insulin signaling and addiction to food, gambling, and drugs. She says, "Research over recent decades has revealed that dopamine and insulin systems do not operate in isolation from each other but instead work together" to orchestrate both the motivation to eat and to calibrate the level of satiety reward from food consumption. She goes on to say, "Insulin signaling has been found to regulate dopomine neurotransmission."[16]

A MAN WHO PUT CHARACTER OVER COMFORT

 Omar, forty-six, an author and bitcoin entrepreneur, had been seen as a patient of our diabetes clinic for six years. A resident of Scarsdale and a devoted husband and father, Omar was the primary caregiver for his two sons. His habit of taking his sons out for burgers and fries after their soccer games had spun his diabetes out of control, and he consulted with the MetaKura team to take action.

He told us that as a kid growing up in New Jersey, he tended to be on his computer to avoid being with other people. His father emigrated from Tunisia, and although this was before 9/11, other kids saw Omar as being different, and he got bullied. With low self-esteem, he said, he probably had anxiety and depression from the age of six. Feeling isolated had an impact on Omar's eating habits. But he told us that he didn't sense the scale of the problem until he went to college. Omar said, "I remember being so hungry. Once I ate a dozen chicken pot pies in one go. I gained forty pounds the first year. Although I managed to take it off, the weight came back on when I was twenty-one."

He was very open about his history of alcoholism and noted that he saw a connection between addiction and his appetite for food. He told us that after a friend committed suicide, he began drinking when he was seventeen because it "took the pain off." His drinking in college escalated: "Once I started consuming alcohol in college, I couldn't stop. Whether I went to a bar at lunchtime or eight p.m., I was the last one to leave. I drank until I passed out. With the beers I drank, I was constantly eating Reuben sandwiches, buffalo wings, or whatever was available."

Sober for ten years, for which he deserves much credit, Omar still struggled with food. He described it as "an overwhelming feeling of craving. I physically can't stop. Nothing else matters. I have absolutely no self-control." As he examined his reaction to food, he noted that there were certain foods that led to this feeling of insatiable hunger more than others.

"If my wife makes chicken parmigiana with pasta, an hour after the meal, I feel tremendously hungry. I don't feel well. It gives me a headache."

Omar also shared with us his hopes for getting his health on track. "I want to be around for my wife and my boys. One of my life principles is to put character over comfort. I want my boys to see that I grew from this experience and could offer an example to the next person."

Clinic Notes

Omar was five foot five and weighed 260 pounds. His father had a triple bypass and later died from complications of heart disease. His father's eighty-seven-year-old sister had heart issues as well. She and both his paternal grandparents had diabetes. Omar's mother had an English-German heritage, and her mother was an alcoholic who died of a heart attack after becoming sober.

Omar has shown tremendous courage in resolving his alcohol addiction. The links between insulin resistance, addiction, binge eating, or drinking are not yet fully understood. But Omar had clearly inherited his insulin-resistant metabolic genes from his father. His fondness for beer led to weight gain and progressively worsening diabetes. This condition was further aggravated by the fast-food feasts he had with his sons. For clients who have a tendency to indulge, a small number (about 10 percent) seem to be able to reward themselves once a month, by allowing one piece of chocolate without going on to consume the whole box. They are also able to eat more widely during regular meals. Not trusting his own food instincts, Omar chose to limit his weekly meal choices to two or three variations.

We recommended that Omar with his Ruby metabolism consume natural food with texture and complexity that required chewing to trigger the release of the most satiety hormones. These include cabbage, Brussels sprouts, bok choy, and cauliflower, as well as select fruits, lean meat, fish, and other protein foods, which are also good choices for their nutritional benefits. There are also benefits to eating some raw food. For example, 53 grams of raw apple can be eaten every minute, compared to eating an apple purée where one can consume 141 grams a minute, or 619 grams a minute for apple juice.[17]

Midway through the MetaKura program, Omar was laid off from work. Rather than reverting to his earlier pattern of despair, Omar began offering counseling to his former colleagues. That decision, he said, resulted in a lifetime journey of personal growth.

Over the next six months, Omar adhered to the same weekly menu except when he was on vacation. He actually found the lack of choice comforting. He reversed his symptoms of diabetes by normalizing his blood glucose (HbA1c 11.2 to 5.5 percent) for the first time in years and shed forty-one pounds as he did so.

THREE PORTRAYALS OF HUNGER DISORDER

Lack of sleep, stress, seasonal changes, exercise, and the types of food we eat are among the many factors that trigger hunger pangs. Overriding these factors are common appetite signal disorders that we frequently encounter.

1. *The midnight marauder:* One of our patients told us that when she stayed at hotels, she would wake up to piles of candy wrappers in the room and chide her husband for raiding the minibar in the middle of the night. He denied it. Later, she found out that she and her nightly tranquilizer were the culprits. Some individuals may wake up at night, comfort their anxiety with a snack, and fall asleep with little recollection of their nocturnal escapades.

   "On Wall Street I worked sixteen hours a day and slept for six hours. I was a restless sleeper who would wake up to eat in the night. But not anymore," said our patient Jill.

2. *The Svengali:* Antonia, a senior executive at a consumer goods company who had been a celebrated chess champion in a Baltic country in her youth, told us that at the end of her workday, before going to her home, she called her husband to tell him to lock up all the chocolate in the house. She could never just eat one piece, she said.

"When I look back, I see a food addiction," recalled another patient, Audrey. "I couldn't just eat one cookie. I ate the whole box. I have two types of hunger, the kind that's like a hole in my stomach that tears into me. In my Svengali moments, usually at night, an inner voice makes me crave bread or cake."

3. *Consumed by cravings:* "Parents should consider teaching children to be sensitive to their appetite signals rather than insisting that they finish all the food on their plate. It only makes the child's appetite grow until it becomes a monster," advised Andrew. "Looking back, I always had a craving for potatoes and bread. The more I ate, the hungrier I became."

A Healthy Appetite in Childhood

Many of our clients have children, and they are very aware of not passing along erratic eating habits at the family table. We have devised some ideas for parents to think about when they are having meals with their kids:

Food portions: Small, frequent meals are prefereable. A UK study found that consuming larger portions at two years of age was associated with more rapid weight gain by the time a child was five years old. Young children who eat larger amounts at each meal are more prone to excess weight than ones who eat more frequently.[18]

Eating slowly: Extend family mealtimes. Among four-and-a-half-year-olds whose mealtimes varied between two minutes and thirty-five minutes, faster meals are associated with a higher energy intake, a higher BMI, and more weight around their tummies than children who ate more slowly.[19]

Exposure to a variety of foods: As they grow, children come to associate specific features of a food, such as its flavor, texture, and appearance, with how full they feel after the meal. They then learn to use these sensory cues to guide meal choices. Introduce your child to a variety of foods and flavors.

Sharing meals: There are the biochemical benefits of "commensality" or sharing meals with others. In a Korean study, married individuals consumed more vegetables, and men and women who lived alone tended to have a higher body mass index and a greater risk for metabolic syndrome.[20] Says Sidney Mintz, professor of anthropology at Johns Hopkins University, "Interaction over food is the single most important feature of socializing. The food becomes the carriage that conveys feelings back and forth." Family meals should be shared—if not every day, then at least a few times a week.

Limiting access to television: This is important not only to help children avoid a sedentary lifetyle but to limit their exposure to the marketing of calorie-dense processed food. Early experience with high-calorie processed foods can increase a child's inclination to favor these foods.

Appealingly packaged snacks and drinks (including the majority of so-called health foods) are irresistible to many because they are comforting, affordable, easy to find, and offer bursts of flavor. Don't be fooled. Closely read the fine print on their ingredient labels. More often than not, these products (including items served in restaurants or food outlets) have been engineered to alter your appetite signals and increase your food cravings. To test our thesis, eliminate all sugars and grains from your diet for three weeks. Then try eating a slice of pizza or a bowl of rice and notice the immediate effect this food has on your energy levels and mental alertness. Hundreds of our patients have chosen to eliminate these "metabolic overload" foods and have calmer, more manageable appetites. You can too.

CHAPTER 6

Gut Reaction: The Power of the Microbiome

The body and its parts are in a continuous state of dissolution and nourishment, so they are inevitably undergoing permanent change.

—Ibn al-Nafis (1213–1288), Arab physician and polymath

The first clue was Eddie's thinning hair.

Eddie, forty-six, is the CEO of a small New York–based luxury goods firm. His type 1 diabetes was diagnosed when he was three years old. Tall, personable, and quick-witted, during the many years that he had been coming to the MetaKura Clinic, he became a father to two daughters and a son.

Recently, Eddie reported feeling tired during the day. He said, "I need hits of caffeine to get through the afternoon. And another thing, I find driving long distances quite challenging. I have to pull over and have my wife take over."

As we investigated further, when asked about his digestion, he remarked, "The usual. Apart from the occasional eruption." Because people with type 1 diabetes are susceptible to other autoimmune diseases and in light of Eddie's digestion issues, we had Eddie tested for celiac disease (an immune disease that causes people to be unable to digest gluten) by evaluating his antibodies.

Sure enough, when we checked for antibodies, Eddie's immunoglobin tests indicated celiac disease (elevated antibody markers in the blood of IgG-1097 and IgA-353). Three years later Eddie's numbers dropped to a normal range of IgG-0.6 and IgA-7.2, respectively. To understand Eddie's story, and how he was able to make positive changes, we will need to take a tour down the alimentary canal.

Every few hours, like a wearied hiker on the Appalachian Trail, the equivalent of four hundred steps are made carrying food over the varied terrain of our digestive tract at a plodding, slow pace. The time needed to traverse the small distance of the alimentary canal (which includes the esophagus, stomach, and intestines) can stretch from thirty-six to over seventy-two hours. At the end of its journey, what began as an exquisitely flavored and desirable object is unceremoniously rubbished. Ambrose Bierce, the American satirist, described the esophagus as the part of the digestive tract that lies between pleasure and business.[1] When pathogens are consumed, the same distance can be crossed at quicksilver speed.

Recently, there has been a sea swell of medical studies asserting that the microorganisms that inhabit our gut—bacteria, fungi, parasites, and viruses—are contributors to weight gain, depression, autism, and other disorders. In 1882, when the Ukrainian-born zoologist Élie Metchnikoff, whose scientific work was at first dismissed as "an Oriental fairytale born in the head of a Cossack,"[2] took up the study of the flora of the human intestine, he established an association between the consumption of fermented milk with increased longevity among rural Bulgarians.[3] Yet by 1907, Metchnikoff noticed "different susceptibilities of people to the harmful effects of microbes. Some can swallow without any evil result, a quantity of microbes which in the case of other individuals would produce a fatal attack of cholera."[4] At the present time, competitive teams of well-funded scientists are attempting to expand Metchnikoff's work to unravel the multichannel conversations of neurons, hormones, and immune cells that occur between the brain and the gut microbiome as they pertain to nutrition, metabolism, pathogen resistance, and brain function.

A HUNDRED TRILLION INHABITANTS

The microbiome is thought of as a community of microorganisms that occupy a well-defined habitat, in this case the gut, which has a distinct effect on the body. In talking about digestion and the microbiome, there are two important factors to consider. First, the microbiota research to date has largely been hampered by an inability to grow and test these same bacteria in laboratory cultures. As a result, most studies have been done in mice. It remains unclear the extent to which experimental findings in mice translate to human outcomes. Harnessing the power of next-generation DNA and RNA–sequencing technology, progress in human studies is nevertheless being made at hurtling speed. Second, and here's the good news, it does not appear that the composition of our microbiomes depends on inherited genes, but it has been acquired through environmental exposures, which means it is possible to effect changes. In a few short weeks, like a seasoned gardener, you can choose the right combination of "plants" for your alimentary flora, manage the pests or sow the right bacteria, and be alert to seasonal changes such as illness and advancing age.

A healthy adult is comprised of about ten trillion human cells. Although they are smaller in size, there are ten times more microbiota than human cells in the body.[5] Together, they collectively weigh about three to four pounds, comparable to the size of the brain. In terms of sheer volume, microbial cells are an unsurpassable superpower. Microbiota eclipse our cells in other ways. While humans have about twenty-five thousand genes, our microbiome has at least five hundred times more. In later adult life, the human gut microbiota goes through changes when a lower diversity of microorganisms and more pro-inflammatory species reside in the large intestine.

Early life is a critical period for establishing a microbial profile for future health. A newborn baby coming from a sterile intrauterine environment acquires its mother's microbiome during the natural birthing process and perhaps even earlier.[6] Contacts with breast skin provide another early source of external microbial bacteria. An infant acquires immune tolerance toward foods and common bacteria via its microbiome. By about two years of age, most children's microbiome stabilizes to a point that their microorganism colonies are similar to that of an adult.[7] Antibiotics, poor diets, and stress in infancy lead to an imbalance in microflora, or dysbiosis, and are associated with immune-related ailments like asthma, celiac disease, and, as our academic research has shown, type 1 diabetes.[8]

From the age of twelve, the bacterial life-forms within us stabilize until their eventual decline in later life. In adults, 60 to 70 percent of the microbiome is stable, with changes occurring based on dietary changes and infections.[9] A high-fiber diet, one rich in vegetables and fruits and low in meat and dairy, is associated with a bacteria called *Prevotella,* while a diet rich in animal fats produced a microbial profile of *Bacteroides*. Rich bacterial variety is associated with lower body weight.[10] And the gut is not only involved with digestion. There is a unique connection between gut function and the brain.

So far, there has not been indisputable proof that microbial messengers are the primary determinants of gut-brain-microbiota interaction. This eloquent, multifaceted, although not entirely well-understood, two-way exchange between the brain and the gut contributes closely to coordination of gastrointestinal activities, and it is also believed to have a profound influence on moods, behavior, learning, and memory. Alterations in the gut-brain axis are associated with anxiety and depression and are more frequently seen in people with insulin resistance.[11] Michael Gershon of Columbia University and others have referred to the gastric or enteric nervous system, which comprises five hundred million neurons, as a "second brain." Fifty percent of the body's dopamine, a neurotransmitter associated with reward and pleasure, is produced in the digestive area, although it cannot cross the blood-brain barrier. Ninety-five percent of serotonin, another signaling molecule associated with appetite, memory, moods, sexuality, and sleep, is also produced by the digestive system. The gut-brain connection was observed by the eleventh-century

Persian physician Avicenna, who wrote in the *Canon of Medicine*, "Mental excitement or emotion; vigorous exercise; these hinder digestion."[12] Today's researchers are beginning to map out this territory, and psychobiotics, or bacteria with positive effects on mental health, are presently being studied for targeted interventions for mental health.[13]

Digestive Dynamos: The Dudes and the Duds

Probiotics like kefir, kimchi, and sauerkraut are live microorganisms that have been shown to confer health benefits. Prebiotics, on the other hand, are nondigestible nutrients found in asparagus, garlic, and tomatoes, among others, that also have beneficial physiological effect. Let's take a closer look at their actions.

>   **Probiotics:** If intestinal bacteria could sensitize the body to insulin and induce us to become leaner, then why not take these bacteria as probiotic supplements? The appeal of this idea is evident in a ballooning patent-rich $35 billion industry for yogurts and kefirs that claim to bring health and balance to digestion and promote weight loss. Unfortunately, the health-related findings behind this industry are replete with unsubstantiated claims. While the body's microbiome flora has not been cultured and expanded artificially (at least not yet), the widely touted lactobacillus, the most common probiotic supplement, has not been shown to promote sustained metabolic health and weight loss. Furthermore, we question the evidence that probiotics containing lactobacilli can survive their passage through the acidic gastric environment stomach to the small intestine for extended periods of time. We agree with Ed Yong, who wrote in *I Contain Multitudes*, "There is no clear evidence that probiotics help people with allergies, asthma, eczema, diabetes...or another disorder in which the microbiome has been implicated. And it is not clear if the touted benefits happen because of changes in the microbiome."[14]

At least two randomized controlled trials have found no effects from probiotic bacteria on human mood or mental health.[15,16]

Prebiotics: They improve digestion and increase bifidobacteria in the human gut, which is thought to protect against pathogens and amplify the body's immune responses. It has been found that prebiotic supplements given to formula-fed babies reduce their episodes of infections in the first six months of life.[17] Two years later, these same prebiotic-fed infants had significantly lower levels of allergies.[18]

At our clinic, we give a big yes to prebiotics and a qualified no to probiotics.

ALIMENTARY INTELLIGENCE

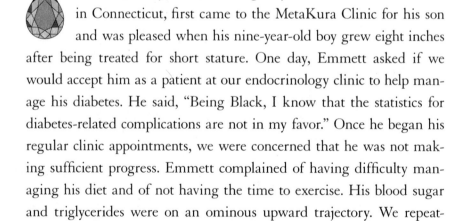 Emmett, forty-three, an elegantly attired economist based in Connecticut, first came to the MetaKura Clinic for his son and was pleased when his nine-year-old boy grew eight inches after being treated for short stature. One day, Emmett asked if we would accept him as a patient at our endocrinology clinic to help manage his diabetes. He said, "Being Black, I know that the statistics for diabetes-related complications are not in my favor." Once he began his regular clinic appointments, we were concerned that he was not making sufficient progress. Emmett complained of having difficulty managing his diet and of not having the time to exercise. His blood sugar and triglycerides were on an ominous upward trajectory. We repeatedly expressed our concern to Emmett that, unless he made significant changes, he might need to take insulin injections to manage his diabetes. Everything changed one day when Emmett phoned the clinic and asked to join the MetaKura metabolism correction program immediately.

"I've just spent a couple of days in the hospital with my younger brother after his kidney transplant," Emmett told us. "He's thirty-eight years old, has diabetes, and had a triple heart bypass. Being in the hospital pushed me over the edge because of my phobias. But it was also a catalyst for me. I know that if I don't act now, I will end up like him."

Emmett suffered from claustrophobia, preferring bridges to tunnels, stairs to elevators. Despite years of back pain, he could not agree to an MRI test even in an open machine. Emmett successfully lost forty-five pounds and two years later has maintained his weight. When we contacted him to share his observations on his metamorphosis, Emmett said, "Being an economist, I'm a numbers guy. Even now, I count my food calories with an app—even though the MetaKura program says I don't have to. It's a big moment for me when I weigh myself every morning. On a day-to-day basis, I could lose or gain two pounds. I measure my walks with my Fitbit. It's like a game I play with myself. A lot of my phobias stemmed from my acute anxiety about my health. Now I'm thrilled to be back in control."

Clinic Notes

Emmett was five foot six and weighed 227 pounds on his first appointment. He said his great-grandmother had become blind due to her diabetes. Despite the family history, he preferred to keep his own diabetes a secret from his family members. He said that his childhood friends teased him for being fat and that his grandparents joked that he emptied their fridge of its leftovers when he visited their home. Emmett said he may have had diabetes in high school because by then he was always thirsty and frequently ran to the bathroom. He was never tested. Emmett had four episodes of kidney stones before he came to the clinic, as well as a genetic predisposition for high calcium levels (his levels were 10.9 to 11.9; normal is 8.6 to 10.3 mg/dL). Two of his children, also clinic patients, shared this trait with him.

Foods that do not cause this spike of insulin include buckwheat, lima beans, chickpeas, red beans, and lentils. We encouraged Emmett to add them to his diet. We, among others, believe that foods or compounds containing soluble complex carbohydrates (prebiotic foods) stimulate the growth of a desirable microbiome and may improve the absorption of calcium and reduce calorie intake. Healthy adults who are fed a prebiotic—inulin found in chicory root, leeks, asparagus, onions, and garlic—experienced less hunger and greater levels of satiety. Inulin shows a range of beneficial effects on gut microflora, lowering blood glucose, and improving immunity. It was noted that with these changes, the levels of GLP-1 in the adults tested were shown to increase.[19] Radishes, green beans, artichokes, and other vegetables fermented in salt brine are also known to possess anti-oxidative and anti-inflammatory properties.

Those Gut Feelings

For those faced with digestive issues, either in the form of a stalled digestion (constipation) or an overactive one, perhaps as a result of a bacterial infection, we recommend certain foods.

To Promote Digestion	To Restrain an Overactive Digestion
Hummus with raw baby carrots or celery	Steamed vegetables
Buckwheat or steel-cut oatmeal (lightly cooked)	Soups to replenish fluids and salts
High-fiber lentil pasta, walnuts, almonds	Avoid fats and oils
Cacao 75% water-based drinks	Plain Greek yogurt, poached eggs
Cabbage or spinach with turmeric	Ginger, mint, and chamomile tea

NATURE'S MAGIC MEDIATORS

Short-chain fatty acids are the unheralded saviors of your digestive health. Although they do not have the sex appeal of caviar, or the faint aroma of Silk Road bazaars evoked by a digestive dynamo like turmeric, and while definitive studies illuminating their actions are eagerly awaited, we think you might need to befriend them. When soluble complex carbohydrates (prebiotics) are consumed, their absorption depends largely on the efficiency of gut microbiota in the large intestine. Once digested, the remnants are reincarnated as three types of short-chain fatty acids.*

Credited with giving us steady sources of 10 percent of our body energy, short-chain fatty acids can help regulate sodium and water absorption. They reduce glucose output by the liver, which is especially helpful for people with diabetes (indeed, such individuals have been reported to harbor decreased numbers of butyrate-producing intestinal bacteria). Additionally, these digestive agents don't let you feel hungry. The presence of short-chain fatty acids activates the intestine to release satiety-inducing peptides, notably the appetite suppressing peptide YY (PYY) and glucagon-like peptide 1 (GLP-1) that result in feelings of fullness. Increased fiber intake diminishes the appetite, improves insulin sensitivity, and reduces body fat accumulation.[20]

Short-chain fatty acids have three additional vital roles. First, they foster tight cellular junctions in the intestinal mucosal barrier to guard against harmful bacteria and toxins. Breaks in the intestinal walls, as the name implies, leads to the putative "leaky gut" syndrome. Second, short-chain fatty acids suppress inflammation-causing cytokines like interleukin 6 (IL-6) and tumor necrosis factor alpha (TGF-α)—elevations of which are common side effects of insulin resistance. Third, these superheroes of digestion also generate increased numbers of regulatory thymus-derived lymphocytes (T-cells), which stabilize the immune system.

A GUT REACTION TO STRESS

At the MetaKura Clinic, we see people with insulin resistance whose chronic stress interferes with their alimentary canal. Jasmine, an affable and self-analytical thirty-nine-year-old, is a director of a New York state psychiatric center. She came to the Meta-Kura Clinic after experiencing years of frustration trying to resolve her

---

* acetate, propionate, and butyrate

autoimmune thyroid disease. Once she understood that her thyroid function had stabilized and that her blood work confirmed her insulin resistance, she quickly began connecting the dots.

"For many years, I had a feeling that something was wrong. One doctor told me that I had problems with my adrenal function. Now finally, it all makes sense. It would be *such* an effort to get myself to work in the mornings. I'd hit a slump around three p.m. On the ride home, I would make lists of all that I wanted to do that evening. Once I got home, I couldn't get off the couch. Nothing would get done," said Jasmine.

Once Jasmine changed her diet, she told us, "It's changed my personality completely. My husband says, 'Who is this person?' I'm smiling on the outside *and* on the inside. A few weeks ago, my husband and I did a 5K run at a community fund-raiser. You know, it's been a long time coming... I've had gastric problems all my life. It was normal for me to have an upset tummy every day. I often have cramps and severe heartburn. I've been on acid reflux medication for twenty-five years."

Staying on the MetaKura diet has helped keep her gastrointestinal issues in check. "My husband and I really notice the difference when I go astray. On Thursday, we went to a friend's place and they only had pizza. I felt sluggish after having a slice. Eating carbs almost makes me feel manic. After those episodes, I am so exhausted I don't want to get out of bed."

Prior to coming to the Clinic, Jasmine was experiencing a lot of stress at work. She was counseling people who were struggling with everything from post-traumatic stress disorders to prolonged mental illness. On top of that, she was dealing with a difficult boss. It was during this challenging time that she also gained extra weight.

To cope, she ate—mostly cake and candy—but it didn't work. "The more I ate, the more I was depressed." Through tears, Jasmine explained, "I've always felt depressed. As a child, I understood it better when my school friends began talking about suicide. I remember thinking of ways in which it would be okay to end my life. As I grew older, I began to reconcile and integrate my two lives as a Brazilian immigrant who had an American childhood. My life got better and better. But I now see so clearly that anxiety is tied to food cravings."

Clinic Notes

Jasmine was five foot two and weighed 207 pounds at her first appointment. She is married and has no children. Her blood work confirmed her insulin resistance and showed a vitamin D deficiency. She was treated for hypothyroid function.

Jasmine's parents are cousins. Her mother and father have diabetes, as do her maternal aunts and uncles. She said that her younger brother is overweight.

Jasmine responded well to the drug metformin. It is widely used by our clinic to improve insulin sensitivity in those with insulin resistance as well as type 2 diabetes. Although the drug is derived from extracts of the leaves of the French lilac plant, it remains unclear whether the beneficial effects are mediated through the microbiome or not. A similar plant-based agent named berberine has long been prescribed by traditional Chinese medical practitioners, but because it has adverse side effects like muscle wasting, we discourage its long-term use.

Jasmine credits the MetaKura program with resolving a number of her medical complaints—years of waking up dizzy with vertigo, wheezing bouts of asthma, and a rash on her leg that continued making reappearances after a jellyfish bite in Aruba. We have repeatedly praised her for her resolve in losing twenty-seven pounds and, more significantly, acting to avoid medical complications later in life.

ULCERS, GASTRITIS, AND PANCREATITIS

The English poet and theologian John Henry Newman said, "Science is knowledge which has undergone a process of intellectual digestion." All too often, we in the medical profession suffer attacks of dyspepsia. Some years ago, Noel addressed a medical conference about an enzyme he had evaluated to diagnose atrophic gastritis for people like Jasmine who have an autoimmune thyroid disease. About half of all women with thyroid disorders such as Hashimoto's or Graves' disease go on to acquire another autoimmune disorder affecting the stomach. Gastric autoimmunity leads to progressive damage (atrophic gastritis) resulting in a failure to absorb dietary iron and vitamin B_{12}. At the end of the presentation, an eminent gastroenterologist handed Noel a note that said "Bullshit!" Later, after the clinical findings were published in a respected journal, he apologized, and we became friends.[21]

Over drinks one evening, our skeptical companion then confessed that in 1982 he had the same initial negative response to the pioneering work of Australians Barry Marshall and Robin Warren. They showed that gastric ulcers were not psychosomatically induced but instead were caused by underlying infectious bacteria. To dramatically prove their hypothesis, Marshall and Warren drank a rancid broth of *Helicobacter pylori* bacteria, and successfully treated themselves for the ensuing ulcers with cocktails of antibiotics. Even after curing hundreds of people, Marshall and Warren's discovery was politely ignored for the next decade, until 2005, when the Nobel committee recognized their work. Gastric ulcers do not occur with increased frequencies in persons who are insulin resistant.

Abdominal Pain

"To interpret abdominal pain requires the best skill of the finest head," wrote Byron Robinson in *The Abdominal and Pelvic Brain*, his 1907 classic in medical literature. Not a few celebrated personalities, Alexis de Tocqueville and Paul Dirac among them, lived almost their entire lives with mysterious stomachaches, despite having access to the best medical care of their times.[22] Nearly in his eighties, Paul Dirac, a brilliant physicist, was frail and had to be admitted to hospital every few months for vitamin infusions to augment his ailing digestion. It was only then, after a lifetime of extreme gastric discomfort, that a friend diagnosed that Dirac had rare deficiency of stomach acid.[23] At the MetaKura Clinic, abdominal ultrasound scans of our patients with insulin resistance occasionally reveal clusters of pebbles or pain-inducing gallstones.

A FIERY BELLY

Yoshiko, sixty-five, recently retired as an engineering project manager and now dedicates her time to pottery, volunteering at a community kitchen, and promoting diversity in schools. Wise, generous, and courageous, Yoshiko is also a dear friend. She was born in Nagoya, Japan, and at the age of eighteen received a scholarship to study in California and decided to live there. There are unmistakable signs that insulin resistance has loomed over generations of her family. Yoshiko's mother and maternal grandmother had Alzheimer's. Her father and all his nine siblings faded away with some form of cancer of the digestive tract. With that family legacy, a physician cousin had warned her to be on high alert for any gastric ailments.

"For twenty years, I had a dull pain in my abdomen caused by gallstones, which got progressively worse," said Yoshiko. "Eventually, I would wake up five or six times at night to change my position." She habitually took medication for acid reflux. As a child, Yoshiko had a severe allergy to milk and eggs that disappeared during puberty and reappeared in raging attacks of seasonal asthma when she moved to the United States. "When I finally opted for surgery to have the gallstones removed, it was simpler than a tooth extraction." Yoshiko smiled. "I had the surgery on a Friday and attended a friend's wedding the very next day."

Gallstones

A number of our clinic's insulin resistant patients are found to have "silent" gallstones, which are hardened, pebble-like collections comprised of cholesterol, bilirubin, and calcium salts that form in the gallbladder. Bile, formed in the liver to break down fats, is stored in a concentrated form in the gallbladder. For 25 percent of adults in the United States, consuming quick-burning sugars found in fruit, starches, and milk accelerates the formation of triglycerides by the liver leading to non-alcoholic fatty liver disease (NAFLD). An inflamed liver, termed non-alcoholic steatohepatitis (NASH), carries a risk of progressing to non-alcoholic cirrhosis for 3 to 12 percent of the country's population.

At times, gallstones may block the outflow of bile into the lumen of the intestine, leading to acute colicky pains in the upper right abdomen just under the rib cage. As with our friend Yoshiko, it is likely to recur and therefore surgical removal of the gallbladder (cholecystectomy) is the definitive solution. Or gallstones can lodge themselves in the bile duct itself. Then bilirubin—a breakdown product of hemoglobin from recycled red blood cells—accumulates in the blood, leading to a jaundiced complexion.

A PEDICAB DRIVER'S DISTRESS

 Pancreatitis, another abdominal complication of insulin resistance that we see from time to time, can be fatal. On a clear wintery night in 2009, we got a call from the hospital that a patient of ours had been admitted to the ICU. Charles, forty-two, is a boyish, blond actor, a film producer, and pedicab driver who divides his time between New York and L.A. Charles had returned to New York City the previous day after a week of filming in Florida, where he was lead actor in an independent film.

Charles said, "The film director had very little money, and I didn't make my dietary needs clear to him. For days, we ate at Arby's and other fast-food places. The night the filming was over, I drank, and drank, and drank sweet frozen drinks and ate pizza. I returned to New York City and spent the next day pedicabbing around Times Square. In the evening, I went to eat at a diner in the Flatiron area. Just as my order of brisket arrived, I felt a massive aching pain shooting down my rib cage. Somehow, I got myself home. I was curled in bed with oceans of sweat pouring off my brow, but I knew what I had to do. Trudging like a snowman in four feet of snow, I got myself to a hospital on Seventh Avenue. They took some X-rays, put me in an ambulance, and rushed me to Lenox Hill Hospital, where I spent two days in the ICU. The memory of the abdominal pain still haunts me."

Clinic Notes

Charles's attack of pancreatitis was acute. The multifaceted metabolic consequences of insulin insensitivity include increased visceral fat or triglycerides in the liver (fatty liver), which may induce inflammation of the pancreas. People with impaired livers may have a dragging pain under the front lower rib cage. Throughout Charles's medical chart, a recurring note appears: "called him to tell him to cut carbs to lower his TG (triglyceride) levels." Since 2007, when we first saw him, his triglyceride levels have bounced between 1,998 and a normal level of 149. Charles was advised to worry less about fat in his diet and much more about cutting out carbohydrates. While in California, he cooked his own food and did a lot better than in New York, where he tended to get in trouble by eating on the fly. Charles's intake of processed food and sugary drinks caused a rise in triglycerides, which led to pancreatic inflammation or pancreatitis. Now he is a lot more vigilant about his diet.

FOOD INTOLERANCE

While 4 percent of the U.S. population has been diagnosed with lactose intolerance, it is estimated that 50 million Americans suffer from some degree of dairy allergy. Found in milk, lactose is a double sugar (a disaccharide) composed of glucose and galactose that requires an enzyme (lactase) in the small intestine to break it down into its two simple sugars. When someone whose body does not produce sufficient lactase drinks milk, lactose is not absorbed properly. When it is fermented in the large colon by the microbiome, it can produce hydrogen and methane gases, causing bloating pains and stomach turbulence.

Babies have normal amounts of intestinal lactase, and those affected lose lactase by two to three years of age, after which they become lactose intolerant.* In the MetaKura program, we view lactose as the sugar that it is, and typically minimize its intake. Be careful not to purchase lactose-free cow's milk, as it still contains the hydrolyzed monosaccharides, which are simple sugars that need to be avoided. Unsweetened almond or nut milk is our preferred choice for most people.

Not by Bread Alone

 Three years after his diagnosis, Eddie, our celiac patient, said, "My blood tests have shown consistent progress with regard to the lowering of my antibodies. Truth be told, it's harder to manage celiac than my diabetes. Especially in the city, I have to be very, very careful of cross-contamination of gluten in any areas where food is served. We always call restaurants in advance. If they ask if I am gluten sensitive or gluten intolerant, they have won me as a loyal customer. I've found that gluten-free cereals tend to have lots of sugar, which isn't great for my diabetes. So I stick to gluten-free bread and carry special buns when I travel to smaller cities. My family is very careful and supportive. I enjoy cooking and have found that most of my favorite recipes that I've collected for the past twenty years—except Chinese stir-fry—can be adapted with gluten-free ingredients."

Like Eddie, Isabel has type 1 diabetes but was a part of the Meta-Kura program for a few weeks before she made her discovery about celiac. Isabel, fifty-one, a single mother and managing director at a multinational financial services company, has been a boisterous and much-loved

---

* The genetic explanation for this lies in an enhancer region that influences regulation of the lactase (LCT) where one dominant allele is associated with adult lactose tolerance.

presence at our clinic for fifteen years. Her daughter Sandra, who is also our patient, has the added complication of the sickle cell trait that affects one in thirteen Black people. On a fall evening five years ago, Isabel was noticeably jittery when she came for her appointment.

Isabel said, "When I woke up from the gastroenterologist's test, they said that I have celiac disease." Then she wagged her finger at us in mock annoyance as she said, "And now that I've joined the MetaKura program, I hope that I don't get overrestricted in food choices. No gluten, no carbs, no bananas. So what am I supposed to eat?"

Many of our patients believe gluten-free diets are healthier and are disappointed when they don't help with weight loss. We generally support minimizing most grains in the diet and strongly urge avoiding rice, although it is gluten-free.

Clinic Notes

The symptoms of celiac disease include abdominal pain and bloating, and are caused by the malabsorption of nutrients induced by eating foods made from certain grain flours—wheat, rye, and barley. Such foods contain a protein called gliadin. People with celiac disease have an abnormal immunological response to gliadin, which reacts to a normal intestinal enzyme named transglutaminase, associated with intestinal inflammation.* Of the 35 to 40 percent of people who carry the predisposing HLA-D genes, only 0.5 to 1 percent develop celiac disease. Once diagnosed, the treatment is avoiding gliadin in the diet.**

Isabel, five foot three, dropped from 173 pounds to 154 pounds over the six months of the MetaKura program, which she now says was easy to follow. Isabel's meal plan included Portobello mushrooms as bun replacements for sandwiches, eggplant crust pizza, and spaghetti squash

---

* The predisposing genes, found on chromosome 6, are certain human leucocyte antigens (HLA-DQ2 and HLA-DQ8).

** In patients suspected of celiac disease, the diagnosis can be made with a blood antibody test, against transglutaminase TTG (IgA type if recent and IgG type if chronic).

with tomatoes and basil. Isabel's immunoglobin tests in September 2015 for celiac disease were clearly elevated, with blood antibody markers IgG 167 and IgA 135+. Two years later, these numbers had dropped to 2 and 5, respectively.

Committing to a sustained exercise program to help Isabel maintain her weight loss was a challenge for her. "I wish that I had an exercise partner," she said. "I don't like gyms," she complained with her customary candor. "There are too many people walking around butt naked as if they were alone at home. I have all the equipment I need at home—ropes, weights, stretchy bands—but I cannot make the time to put them to use." We struck a deal with Isabel that she use walking for exercise, and she happily walks four or five miles a day.

The steady, uneventful journey of food through the alimentary canal is one of the most persuasive barometers of the health of your metabolism. While it can be a downright challenge for some, as we have shown, solutions abound. Lin Yutang, the Chinese philosopher who famously said that the wisdom of life was the elimination of nonessentials, was even more explicit when he said, "Happiness for me is a good digestion." We agree.

CHAPTER 7

Fat Cells: Exquisitely Designed Hubs of Energy?

[The body is] a marvelous machine...a chemical laboratory, a powerhouse. Every movement, voluntary or involuntary, full of secrets and marvels!

    —Theodor Herzl, playwright and political activist

Just as Charles Darwin elevated earthworms to "living ploughs that nourish the soil," fat cells are enjoying a reputational renaissance. Once considered mere repositories of dietary excess, fat cells have earned newfound respect as exquisitely designed mini-hubs of the metabolism. Fat cells have a hyperactive stealth existence as they silently dispatch lipid-signaling molecules that bring order to the body's busily trafficked pathways.

Present in plants, animals, and microorganisms, lipids are insoluble in water and include fats, waxes, oils, and hormones. Also called adipocytes or lipocytes, they gather to buttress the semipermeable walls of cellular membranes. From this vantage point, fat cells interact with messenger molecules to control our appetite, blood sugar equilibrium, energy metabolism, and immune responses. They are the body's primary energy reservoirs. With flirtatious flair, these lipid-filled vacuoles also regulate our carnal cravings—steroid sex hormones like estradiol and testosterone are synthesized from cholesterol (a lipid). Only now are we beginning to unravel why even small changes in lipid structures can have profound effects on our vital body functions and risk for disease.

When cell sensitivity to insulin deteriorates and ever more levels of the hormone are needed to protect vital physiological needs, a Shakespearean "misshapen chaos of well-meaning forms" ensues.[1] The balance between hunger and satiety hormones in the brain's hypothalamus is disrupted, which invariably leads to a greater appetite. In the gut, internal inflammatory markers become hyperactive and accelerate health-related complications. Insulin's effectiveness in neatly storing fat in adipose tissue declines and long chains of fatty acids begin to populate the bloodstream and obstruct the liver. As the levels of lipotoxicity (lipid poisoning) accrue in the metabolism, this can lead to diabetes and other chronic disease.

Beehive-like clusters of lipid cells are part of the body's ever-present connective tissue that protects our organs along with bones, ligaments, and tendons. The average infant is born with 4 billion fat cells, known as adipocytes. This number increases to 10 to 40 billion in lean people and 50 to 100 billion in heavy individuals. Body mass increase, which makes cells larger, is called hypertrophy.

Noel's earliest insights on disturbances in fat metabolism came during his formative years as a physician, working at London's Great Ormond Street Hospital. There he had the honor of working with Dr. Otto H. Wolff, a towering, genteel man who often invited his colleagues home for dinner followed by chamber music. In an unforgettable series of presentations, he impressed his postdoctoral students with studies being done at Rockefeller University that showed that a person's number of fat cells may decrease during periods of weight loss, but except for extreme cases of weight gain, the number of fat cells remains unchanged after puberty for life.[2]

Between the ages of five and six, some children begin to experience an increase in the *quantity* of fat cells (hyperplasia), or what is termed "the fat rebound."[3] As a precautionary note for parents, a Korean nationwide study, one of many such studies, found that a child considered chubby during the rebound phase is 30 percent more likely to remain so in adolescence and adulthood than a child of average weight.[4]

It has been suggested that an adult woman with 20 percent of her body weight as fat tissue could survive for thirty days without food.[5] This was borne out by archaeologist Donald Grayson of the University of Washington. He studied the female survivors of the infamous Donner Party, a group of nineteenth-century pioneers stranded in the Sierra Nevada by a harsh winter in 1846, where, purported cannibalism notwithstanding, more women than men survived. "Females have greater surface body fat that protects them from the cold," Grayson pointed out. In addition to their tendency to work more collaboratively, he added, women are also able to burn less energy, an evolutionary adaptation to enhance reproduction.[6,7]

In 1947, Jean Vague, a Marseilles-born French endocrinologist, published a paper. He observed that in android (male) forms of excess weight, the accumulation of visceral fat in the abdominal region was associated with a threefold increased risk for cardiovascular disease. The gynoid (female) type of overweight, Vague wrote, favored fat stores in the gluteo-femoral region (hips and thighs) and was less harmful. At the time, Europe was still in a postwar gloom and Jean Vague's insights, which have since been corroborated, were ignored by the scientific community for the next three decades.[8]

Fat cells, or adipocytes, which have a mind-bending range, are identified by a highly stratified caste system based on:

- their location—subcutaneous (below the skin) or visceral (in the abdominal cavity)
- whether they store energy (triglycerides)
- whether they build cells, tissues, and hormones (cholesterol)
- their appetite-regulating chemical messengers (leptin and adiponectin)
- their color (white, brown, or beige).

The Undercover Agents of Fat Metabolism

Learn the language of fat:

Adipocytes: fat cells.

Cholesterol: a waxy, fatty substance found in all animal cells that is integral to countless bodily processes.

High-density lipoprotein cholesterol (HDL): considered the "good" cholesterol. High levels are cardioprotective.

Low-density lipoprotein (LDL): considered the "bad" cholesterol because high levels are risk factors for arteriosclerosis, coronary heart disease, and stroke.

Triglycerides: three fatty acids (linked to glycerol) that are produced by the liver as by-products of the fructose and sucrose present in simple carbohydrate foods.

White fat: what we think of as bodily fat, and the body's source of energy.

Brown fat: tissue that converts food to heat and energy.

Beige fat: a hybrid of white and brown fat that may be able to activate white fat to convert to energy.

Subcutaneous fat: the fat found beneath the skin.

Visceral fat: the fat found in the lining of the abdominal cavity.

Fatty acids: the building blocks of body fat derived from foods: saturated, monounsaturated, polyunsaturated, and trans fats, and when artificially solidified from oils into trans fats.

Leptin: the appetite-suppressing fat cell–derived hormone. The more body fat you have, the more leptin you produce. Insulin resistant people become leptin resistant.

Adiponectin: a fat cell–derived hormone that helps muscles and the liver become more sensitive to insulin.

WHEN FAT GETS IN THE WAY

"I don't like looking in the mirror anymore," admits Max. An early class of antiviral drugs called protease inhibitors enabled this eighty-five-year-old lawyer to arrest his AIDS syndrome many years ago. An unfortunate side effect of these medications is the destruction of the fat cells that produce the hormone leptin. As a result, Max has minimal subcutaneous fat, the dominant form of body fat found beneath the skin, which gives his face a flattened look.

"After almost dying of whooping cough as a baby, I was skinny until the age of twelve," Max recalls, "but that did not last. From then on, I tried all kinds of diets to keep my weight down until I was diagnosed with HIV at the age of fifty-seven." Despite his lean, youthful physique, tests showed that Max presented the full range of fat, or lipid, metabolism gone haywire. Max's insulin resistance caused his visceral fat, which is found in the lining of the abdominal cavity, to grow in proportions similar to someone with a huge belly. His liver was slightly enlarged, and his triglyceride levels hovered high above the normal range.

People who are born with a rare congenital absence of fat cells have a condition called lipodystrophy. With the absence of the appetite-suppressing hormone leptin, they are known for their hearty appetites. Now, because triglycerides (blood lipids) cannot be stored normally, they accumulate fat in the liver, pancreas, blood, and muscle tissue. Often this causes a kind of lipotoxicity, and with it, a severe form of insulin resistance. In a spectacular turnaround, when such individuals are treated with leptin injections, all these problems are resolved, including their symptoms of diabetes.

Banting's Unanswered Cry for Help

In 1869, a desperate London undertaker penned a plea that has been largely unanswered across the decades. In his *Open Letter on Corpulence,* William Banting wrote, "Among the parasites that plague us all, I cannot think of any more distressing than being overweight…[It] seems to me very little understood or properly appreciated by the faculty [medical professionals] and the public generally, or the former would long ere [before] this have hit upon the cause for so lamentable a disease, and applied effective remedies."

Banting's 150-year-old lament over the public and medical attitude toward the heavier members of society, in his words, "injudicious indulgence in remarks and sneers, frequently painful in society, and which, even on the strongest mind, have an unhappy tendency," are less archaic than his English. Compare his statement with one that Alice, a thirty-year-old architect, recently expressed to us: "It [excess weight] almost felt like having a disability. The bias against fat people is the last discrimination against a person that isn't protected against by law."

Every day we encounter people, whether at our clinic, or in parks, airports, and cafés, who are stymied by their unwanted body fat. We want to approach them and say, "It's not your fault. More than likely, you have insulin resistance and here are all the actions you can take to bring it under control."

A Gifted Child's Dangerous Predicament

On Palm Sunday, light through the stained glass falls like a blessing on the congregation gathered at Inwood's Our Lady Queen of Martyrs Catholic Church. Worshippers, mostly from the Dominican Republic, fill the pews and weave palm fronds into crosses. At the podium, a silvery-voiced member of the choir raises her palms upward to lead the first hymn. "Being part of the choir is my passion," says forty-two-year-old Gloria. "I'm a soprano, though I'm very shy about singing solo parts. My faith is the motor that drives my life." After a sixteen-year career as a computer programmer for a leading firm of naval architects, today she helps design highly advanced ships and submarines for navies the world over.

Gloria's daughter, Gaby, attends Manhattan's Gifted and Talented

Anderson School and plays the violin, flute, guitar, and trumpet. She is equally talented as an artist. Gaby's father, Fernando, first raised the alarm about their thirteen-year-old daughter's weight problem. His four full-figured sisters all suffer from chronic thyroid imbalances.

"Gaby will have a big *quinceañera*," declares her mother, referring to a celebration of a fifteen-year-old Latina's transition into womanhood that features sparkling tulle dresses, DJs, and bands. Gloria adds, "We hope she loses her puppy fat by then. After seeing Dr. Maclaren, we have drastically changed Gaby's diet."

Clinic Notes

As mentioned previously, following the final pubertal rebound phase, which occurs at an average age of sixteen, the number of fat cells remains fixed for life. Heavier individuals who have been chubby children have more fat cells (adipocytes) than lean people, and, importantly, that number of cells is forever. This is true even if, at a future date, an individual successfully loses half their body weight by dieting or by bariatric surgery. In fact, when remeasured two years after bariatric surgery, the fat cells are leaner, but there is no decrease in their numbers.[9]

Gaby's maternal great-grandmother and grandmother had insulin-dependent diabetes. Although she is now elfin in appearance, Gaby's mother weighed 130 pounds as an eleven-year-old in her Dominican village. Fernando, Gaby's father, carries 190 pounds on his five-foot-six frame. It is our clinical impression that in newborns such as Gaby who tend to be smaller by one to two pounds than the norm for their gestational age, genetically inherited insulin-related metabolic imbalances are more commonly passed down from the mother's family. Mothers may fret about their baby's slender limbs during infancy and early childhood, only to have matters take a dramatic turn with the onset of puberty.

When a child is about eight or nine, the adrenal glands, which rest on top of the kidneys, go into a pubertal change called adrenarche. A feature of plump children with insulin resistance is premature pubarche, the first appearance of underarm and pubic hair. This early aspect of puberty is often accompanied by pink "stretch marks," or striae, on the groin and shoulders. Gaby's initial examination confirmed that she had such telltale stripes and whorls on her upper arms. Described as a "neuro-immuno-cutaneous-endocrine network," skin striae signal an excess of cortisol, a steroid hormone necessary for managing stress, metabolic, and cardiovascular functions. These striae are pink at first and later fade to the child's skin color. When a twenty-four-hour cortisol output in the urine of such children and young adults is measured, the levels are often elevated. Gaby's initial assessment and blood work showed that her body weight, with a BMI over 30, was of clinical concern.

Gaby's good cholesterol level (high-density lipoprotein, or HDL) was permanently suppressed, leaving her at risk for atherosclerosis (hardening of the arteries), heart disease, or a stroke later in life. Her triglyceride level was elevated due to the exaggerated insulin levels flooding her liver. This damaging combination instructed Gaby's body to produce cascades of triglycerides in her abdominal viscera, liver, muscles, and even in her blood. Of most serious concern, her blood glucose levels indicated that she was in the process of developing type 2 diabetes, placing her at risk for complications such as kidney failure. Fortunately, the development of type 2 diabetes can be halted. With her high insulin levels, the level of protein in her urine (a normal microalbumin creatinine range is less than 15, and Gaby was at 362) already indicated early kidney damage.* We could see dangerous health threats ahead for this gifted child.

----

* Fat cells, or adipocytes, release leptin and cortisol. Cortisol is a highly active form of the hormone, secreted by the adrenal glands, whereas cortisone is a form that is more inactive. These two forms coexist in equilibrium. With insulin resistance, enzymes in the body's visceral fat instigate an increased ratio of cortisol to cortisone secretion. There are many clues that suggest that adrenal corticoids may be co-conspirators in weight gain. Paradoxically, the cortisol blood levels are typically not elevated but are often, in fact, found to be normal or low, the reason being that the majority of cortisol, when carried by a protein that is highly mobile in the blood plasma, corticosteroid binding globulin (CBG) is not biologically available or active. The effect of low levels

Tactfully but forcefully, we spelled out for Gloria the risks Gaby faced, concentrating on the lifelong changes she needed to make to counter her daughter's inherited profile. Immediate intervention was essential to avoid a cascade of medical problems.

Our recommendation for Gaby was a diet of high-protein meals with non-starchy vegetables, such as leafy greens, and fruit that is low in sugars, such as berries. Moreover, the family had to join Gaby on her meal plan. We also urged that Gaby exercise daily, preferably by engaging in team sports or dancing, supplemented by walking. Gloria solemnly agreed to change Gaby's diet to improve the health prospects of her only child.

Cholesterol Deserves Our Gratitude

The human brain is the most cholesterol-rich organ (adult brains average approximately 20 percent of the cholesterol in the body) where the waxy molecule ably assists in the formation of synapses and dendrites.

 Audrey, sixty, is the associate dean at a well-regarded New York university. The first clues to her insulin resistance were her skin tags, pearls of extra skin that dotted her cheeks and neck. She weighed 167 pounds at a height of five feet seven inches and wore a size 14 dress. "I want to lose fifteen pounds and my belly fat," Audrey said on her first visit to the MetaKura Clinic. Her tangerine dress picked up the orange in her multicolored vintage eyeglass frames.

Audrey grew up in Far Rockaway, Long Island. Her father left the family when she was eight and had no contact with her thereafter, so she has no knowledge of her paternal family history. Of her mother, she said, "I now realize [she] had a personality disorder and was given to mood swings and rages. I was not a star student, especially with math, and probably had an attention disorder. Growing up in a community where

---

of CBG is that bioavailable levels of cortisol are increased, even when cortisol levels measured in blood samples are found to be low.

every kid aspires to be a lawyer or doctor, not being an academic achiever haunts me to this day. I felt a rung below the others."

Audrey was "very skinny" through third grade, but when she hit puberty, she became ten pounds overweight. "I had a lot of turmoil in my head," she said.

Audrey recalled that her grandmother carried her weight in her stomach. Her mother was slim, smoked two packs a day, and died of lung cancer at age fifty-eight. She had an eccentric uncle, a scholarly linguist and a hoarder, who lived alone and weighed over two hundred pounds. Her brother, a well-known neurosurgeon in Florida, has maintained a trim presence through his adult years.

The mother of three, Audrey gained close to forty pounds during her second pregnancy. "When I look back, I see a food addiction, as I couldn't just eat one cookie. I ate the whole box," she said. "I have two types of hunger, the kind that's like a hole in my stomach that tears into me, and then my hardest moments, usually at night, when an inner voice makes me crave bread or cake." After her third child was born, Audrey lived on a meager diet of coffee, tuna salad, and chicken wings, under five hundred calories a day. It was unsustainable, however. "I couldn't do that anymore," she said.

Audrey's older son has struggled with addiction and has a "beer belly." Her youngest son grew chubby in the fourth grade but lost one hundred pounds in his senior year in high school and had to be treated for anorexia. "I see such powerful patterns repeating themselves in my family. Genes have a huge impact on who you are."

Clinic Notes

Audrey's labs showed that she had abnormal cholesterol levels and confirmed that she had disturbances in her metabolism.

For many with inherited insulin imbalances, especially those who are not athletically inclined, adolescence is when the body's struggle with weight make its first appearance. As this occurs appetite signals get confused and altered. Audrey's skin tags were an additional indicator of elevated insulin in the blood. Her uncontrollable food urges also indicated a metabolic imbalance.

Over the course of more than a year, Audrey's triglycerides improved, as did her energy levels. For people like Audrey, the risk of atherosclerosis is heightened by the combination of high triglycerides and low HDL. This occurs when the individual also happens to inherit a secondary genetic condition that is strongly familial—hypercholesterolemia: an elevation of "bad" cholesterol (low-density lipoprotein [LDL]). Her weight loss pattern was established. Weigh-ins at three-month intervals showed her weight dropping from 167 pounds to 160, 150, 149, and then 147 pounds, and then returning to 148 and finally 150 pounds. This small reversal was thanks to her long daily commute from Manhattan to Far Rockaway in Long Island, which resulted in her eating dinner after eight p.m. Audrey looks young for her years and is so pleased with her new weight that we are confident she will change her meal schedule and maintain her weight loss indefinitely.

AN ODE TO THE LIVER

You raise
And gather
The threads and the grams
Of life, the final
Distillate,
The intimate essences.
—Pablo Neruda, "Ode to The Liver,"
The Elemental Odes

In 2008, the medical journal *Liver International* described a chance sunset encounter in the early 1950s on a beach in Isla Negra, Chile, between Toronto-based physician Hector Orrego and his fellow Chilean, acclaimed poet Pablo Neruda. A man of prolific intensity who penned 3,500 pages of poetry, Neruda reveled in his contradictions as a celebrated diplomat and a political pariah in exile, a towering icon of Latin American intellect and, at heart, an average Joe. It was in the latter spirit that he undertook to write three volumes called *The Elemental Odes* published between 1954 and 1957. According to Professor Marco Arrese, Neruda asked Dr. Orrego to suggest a body part he could include in his collection. Orrego, a liver disease specialist, gave Neruda a series of tutorials on "how the organ resembles a laboratory that modifies everything and maintains the chemistry of the body, how the liver detoxifies, metabolizes and forms every class of substance indispensable for other organs of the body to function, including the brain."[10] Neruda's odes appeared in his friend Miguel Otero Silva's Caracas-based newspaper *El Nacional.* Interestingly, they ran not in the literary supplement but rather on the news pages, where they were read by multitudes of new poetry lovers.

The liver produces triglycerides as the major component of very low-density lipoprotein (VLDL), a complex lipid. Another feature for people with insulin resistance is lipolysis, in which a steady stream of free fatty acids (FFAs) is released from their adipose (fat) stores. Over time, with increased liver enzymes, the Greek names take over: steatohepatitis, (*steat* means "solid fat") or scarring, known as fibrosis or cirrhosis (*kirros,* red-yellow) of the liver.

In our opinion, before prescribing statin drugs, doctors should always recommend low-carbohydrate diets to lower triglyceride levels as a primary course of action. Statins should not be suggested unless the individual's "bad," or LDL, cholesterol is also raised.

Dyslipidemia, in which levels of lipids hover above or sink below the "normal" range, is an important risk factor for coronary disease and stroke.[11] High-density lipoprotein (HDL), which inhibits inflammation and benefits immune responses, was considered a protective form of cholesterol that reduced the risk for cardiovascular disease. More recently, this assertion has been questioned, and HDL's effect on clearing plaques from the arteries may be more complicated than previously thought.[12]

FATS: A PALETTE OF EARTH TONES

In terms of their bodily benefits from temperature regulation to energy production, brown adipose cells found in all mammals far outshine white fat cells. So beneficial are these brown cells that scientists are immersed in far-reaching studies on how to transform white adipose tissue to beige—to create islands of brown fat cells amidst a white expanse. Intense exercise is being carefully studied for its ability to transform the structure of fat cells.

There are three hues of fat cells. White energy-storing fat adipose tissue (WAT) that cushions our waist, hips, and thighs and releases fatty acids for energy. A precious dollop of brown adipose tissue (BAT)—an average of fifty grams (1.7 ounces)—that remains constant through life converts food to heat and energy. In cold weather, using a process of thermogenesis, brown adipose tissue creates heat to maintain body temperature. A recent discovery is that humans have the capacity to create brown-like adipocytes within the white adipose tissue (WAT) called beige adipocytes. These cells burn energy and nutrients at a high rate, and their presence coincides with improved metabolic profiles and blood sugar control.[13] Beige fat is being busily researched for its "plasticity," its ability to activate white fat cells with energy-burning mitochondria. In mice studies, which may or may not be duplicated in humans, negative energy (fewer calories consumed than are burned), as well as exposure to cold, were seen to change gut microbiomes, which in turn accelerated the conversion of beige cells.[14]

Our patient Margherita used strenuous exercise to increase her beige fat and was able to overcome depression, end her cycle of migraines, reboot her energy levels, and restore her metabolism. Margherita speaks fondly of her hometown on the Hudson. "Nyack is a river town. It gets in your blood," she says with pride. "There's an artsy vibe—Edward Hopper had a home here, as did the actress Helen Hayes—but it's also home to miscreants and ne'er-do-wells. There's a faint undercurrent of intrigue."

She shows photos of her three personas over the decades: the fetching, slender, dark-haired bride in her twenties, her lively eyes full of promise. Then a three-generational portrait in her thirties, with her petite mother, her tawny-haired eight-year-old daughter, Dylan, and herself, thirty pounds heavier and offering a reluctant smile. Her forearms are more prominent, her black dress seems fuller, and she has the suggestion of an extra chin. Finally, in her forties, she is running triumphantly across the finish line of a marathon event. Sitting in our office, she is, at forty-four, slim enough to model her wedding dress, her radiance restored.

"Dr. Maclaren was straightforward that I had a genetic inheritance from my father," she says. "My dad was athletic and vigilant about his diet. Whenever we traveled—I remember trips to Paris and Jerusalem—we would have breakfast together after he'd been up at dawn, walking for hours to scope out the city. Yet he died of a stroke in his sixties. I knew that if I did not confront my insulin resistance with diet and exercise, I was on course for medical complications."

When Margherita started our program, her husband, Alex, suggested that they both follow her new dietary regimen. That helped her enormously, though predictably, he (being insulin sensitive) lost twice as much weight as she did in the first two months.

Clinic Notes

On her first visit, Margherita complained of chronic fatigue, frequent migraines, and a low-functioning thyroid. At five feet one inch tall, she weighed 154 pounds, and had been restricting her diet to 1,500 to 1,700 calories a day. By her next visit, Margherita told us she had enrolled in a boot camp workout regimen three times a week. We cautioned her that extreme forms of exercise can lead to the urge to compensate the body with calorie-rich foods, but Margherita was very compliant with her diet and soon began running marathons.

Margherita initially lost a few pounds. We then introduced medication, which she calls her "magic pills," to regulate her insulin, and she lost nine pounds in three months. Two years later, her weight has stabilized at 137 pounds.

We cautioned Margherita to keep a close eye on Dylan, who was delivered by Cesarean section. Evidence is quickly gathering that babies who don't pass through the birth canal have a 13 percent higher risk of excess weight gain later in life, because they have not been exposed to the mother's protective microbiome. Margherita adds, "Now we watch Dylan carefully and hope she won the genetic lottery. So far, so good."

Fat cells have myriads of crucial contributions to our metabolism, from cognition, sexuality, appetite, and body temperature control. Growing scientific evidence suggests that colonies of beehive-like lipid cells also host immune cells, stem cells, and neurons. Many of their secrets are yet to be revealed.

CHAPTER 8

Energy: Speed, Strength, Movement, and Agility

Sometimes you will do something simply because of the magic of the creative spirit. I would argue that at times, the body achieves a movement beyond your wildest dreams.

—Michelle Dorrance, tap dancer and choreographer

Speed, strength, agility, and flexibility inform the MacArthur Fellowship–winning dancer Michelle Dorrance's wondrous ability to dazzle audiences with a heart-stopping combination of movements. As her feet joyfully improvise steps, sounds, and rhythms, a fine-tuned network of cell signaling in her muscles can choose between glucose and fat as energy sources. In the case of Adrian, a cheering audience member with insulin dysfunction, nutrients are not fed or cleared from his muscle tissue efficiently. His body's flexibility to choose between alternate energy sources is impaired.[1] This "metabolic storm" leads to an overriding sense of fatigue. Fear not, we say to people like Adrian, we have a miraculous potion. Exercise offers a high-speed solution to clearing up these congested pathways and adding new energy transporters, thus enhancing the uptake of glucose in the same tired muscle tissue by *fiftyfold*.[2]

THE MAKING OF HIGH-PERFORMANCE ATHLETES

In 2013, Dr. Justin Roberts, previously at the University of Hertford-shire, now at the Cambridge Center for Sport and Exercise Sciences, Anglia Ruskin University, in the United Kingdom, ran a study in which he invited around one hundred male and female recreational athletes between the ages of eighteen and fifty-five to train for their first iron-distance triathlon. Dr. Roberts designed a nine-month training program for his newly energized volunteers and later traveled with his team to the Barcelona Challenge Triathlon. He told us, "It was a very challenging event. Weather conditions were not great leading into the event, with torrential rain on the day." Torrential rain notwithstanding, from the original cohort in this study who completed the training, an impressive 85 percent swam nearly two and a half miles in challenging sea conditions, cycled 112 miles in the downpour, and then completed a draining twenty-six-mile run.

The nine-month preparation for the race, Dr. Roberts said, focused on the three core components of triathlon: swim, bike, run. He designed short and focused fitness routines during the week and longer, slower ones at weekends. Interspersed with this, he also included weekly functional strength-training exercises to support preparations.

When we asked how the participants developed the mental tough-ness to complete the races, Dr. Roberts responded, "The training was designed to gradually progress and extend each participant's comfort zone (in terms of race distances). The majority of people therefore likely went into the event with the belief that they could complete the race because of their knowledge of what they had put into their training." An important outcome of the study, Dr. Roberts said, was the degree of human adaptability the team witnessed among people who began their training with low to average athletic profiles. Now, seven years later, many of these amazing participants have continued to maintain their fitness and interest in exercise.

Interestingly, he added, "In our lab, we assess exercise metabolism based on expired air analysis. Essentially, when we exercise, we use both fat and carbohydrates for fuel. The higher the intensity of the exercise, the greater reliance on carbohydrates to supply energy demand. At low to moderate intensities, people generally burn fat at about 0.1 to 0.6 grams per minute and around one or two grams of carbs per minute. As the intensity increases, cell metabolism favors glucose or insulin-regulated metabolic pathways, so fat oxidation has to decrease.

"For less active individuals, we have observed in other studies a degree of metabolic inflexibility where participants rely on carbohydrate metabolism very early on into exercise (and hence very low at oxidation rates). Improving this metabolic flexibility could be very important to health and active aging. As such, we are aiming to continue research in this area."

Martin Gibala, professor and chair of the Department of Kinesiology at McMaster University and author of *The One-Minute Workout,* believes that so-called superhuman athletes are born, not made. He explains, "In my personal view, the elite performer has a genetic predisposition. This might be a larger heart or greater cardiac output. Optimal training will allow you to get the most of what you've been given by your parents."

In terms of the balance between energy intake and energy expense, you may not know that resting energy expenditure (REE), or the energy required to sustain our bodies during periods of rest, is *higher* in people who are overweight because it takes more energy to support a larger body mass.[3] Among individuals of similar age, sex, height, and weight, there can be a variance of 80 percent in REE based on differences in body weight and body fat, or to phrase it differently, in lean body mass. An important aspect of the intersection of weight loss and exercise is that after a period of weight loss, increasing skeletal muscle (muscle attached to bones) with regular exercise results in a higher resting energy expenditure and helps to avoid a weight rebound.[4] With six weeks of endurance training, the size of muscle fiber and the number of mitochondria present in skeletal muscle can improve by 6 to 8 percent.[5]

CONGESTED ENERGY PATHWAYS

Sadly, a majority of our clinic patients, like Sylvia, feel as though they are living in an eternal energy crisis. As a child, Sylvia danced at a studio affiliated with the Joffrey Ballet until she was told that she could not be a prima ballerina because of her height of four feet ten inches.

"By the age of six or seven, no one at school wanted me on their team because of my height. I've been teased about it my entire life and now carry a bag of heels wherever I go. I learned that it was best if people underestimated me. I taught myself to work harder than anyone else. Eventually, I began to get recognition through my results." Now she is one of the first women legislators of Puerto Rican origin to be elected in the New York tristate area.

Sylvia came to the clinic because of recurrent episodes of feeling tired and confused. "There are days when I just hit a wall," Sylvia admitted. "I'm a different person when I have low blood sugar. I panic and cannot think clearly as I start spiraling down. It may happen after an eighteen-hour day at the state legislature or at my district office, especially when I don't eat or hydrate enough."

Sylvia's strategy was to carry a small bag of macadamia, cashew, or almond nuts with her every day. "If I start dipping low, I will shove the whole lot in my mouth and wait for a few minutes."

When asked about her overall health, Sylvia told us, "To tell you the truth, I've never *not* felt tired. Lots of doctors have told me that the problem is in my head."

Clinic Notes

Sylvia's maternal grandmother was five foot three, had type 1 diabetes, and died at the age of fifty-seven of a heart attack. She told us that her maternal grandfather was "beyond paranoid" and spent his last years in a bedroom with the window shades lowered. Her mother, a retired librarian, is four feet ten inches tall. She has frequent headaches, and throughout Sylvia's childhood, she had to lie down in the early evenings due to exhaustion. Sylvia's younger sister has weight problems. Her father was in good health until he suddenly died of a brain aneurysm, she said; she was estranged from his relatives, so she was not aware of her paternal family's medical history.

We gave Sylvia a glucose monitor in order to test herself when she felt that her blood sugar was low (hypoglycemia). Sure enough, when these episodes occurred, her levels were below the low end of the range of 70 mg/dL (normal blood sugar levels are less than 100 mg/dL during fasting and less than 140 mg/dL two hours after eating). Because Sylvia said that her mother also experienced outbursts of agitation caused by low blood sugar, and because both mother and daughter were of below average height, we suspected a deficiency of growth hormone (GH), which helps maintain blood sugar. By building her muscle and bone strength with exercise, she could draw on these newly created amino acids to stabilize her blood sugar. Sylvia began a forty-five-minute workout, five days a week. She also enrolled in yoga classes and worked with a personal trainer twice a week. After her blood work confirmed the growth hormone deficiency, we advised Sylvia to give herself subcutaneous growth hormone injections. Four months later, she reported that her strength and energy had improved. Best of all, Sylvia said, she had fewer episodes of hypoglycemia. She brought her mother to the Clinic, who was then treated with a similar regimen and was pleased with her positive results.

Two years later, it became clear that Sylvia's symptoms had recurred, as she had worsening energy levels. After repeating a full metabolic study, Sylvia was found to be low in L-carnitine, a protein produced in the body by amino acids synthesized by vitamin C and found in red meat with smaller amounts in avocados and beans.

As mentioned earlier, most of the energy generated by our bodies is produced inside the thousands of organelles or structures called mitochondria that are present in all of our cells—with the exception of red blood cells. We humans could not have evolved without their energy-fueling presence. Mitochondria have their own genetic system, which is inherited in all mammalian species through the mother's egg cell. Mitochondrial DNA is circular like the DNA of bacteria and has been compared to chloroplasts, the structures within plant cells and green algae that help convert energy from sunlight into food for the plant. Evolutionary evidence suggests that these chloroplast organelles were also once free-living bacteria. A theory proposed by the evolutionary biologist Lynn Margulis is that as early as 1.45 billion years ago, mitochondria arose from a bacterial invasion of membraned cells, long before humans were conceived from multicellular precursor life-forms.[6] From an evolutionary perspective, mitochondria offered the advantage of being able to efficiently create life-giving molecules, called ATP (adenosine triphosphate) by metabolizing carbohydrates, amino acids, and lipids and other foods through aerobic respiration.[7]

Sylvia's deficiency in L-carnitine is significant because in human metabolism, carnitine is a carrier protein that transports lipids called free fatty acids into mitochondria so that they can produce energy at a cellular level. This energy takes the form of ATP, which drives cell activities like muscle contractions or nerve signals. ATP has been called the body's energy currency, as it is also made with glucose. Carnitine is vital for the metabolism of plants, mammals, and even some bacteria. When tested, Sylvia was found to have a markedly low level of this essential protein, and we advised her to take supplements. Carnitine deficiency can be genetic, as was the case with Sylvia and her mother, or diet related, which is more common in vegans.

One reason that so many of our patients have chronic fatigue–like symptoms is that insulin resistance is associated with mitochondrial dysfunction.[8] Aside from getting their insulin back in balance, if they have deficiency in carnitine, then supplementation is recommended.

On average, skeletal muscle tissue accounts for between 40 and 50 percent of body mass, and perhaps because it is highly adaptable, it is a central organ that is impaired in insulin dysfunction. Multiple strategies are in play to source the body's energy needs. In the first phase, dietary glucose stored as glycogen in the liver is converted to ATP (which as you will remember feeds the mitochondria in your cells). Liver glycogen replenishes glucose circulating in the blood, while muscle glycogen is reserved for its own local use by its cells.

In evolutionary terms, muscle glycogen gave humans an emergency energy reservoir to escape predators. Muscles evolved to give us the endurance capacity required to flee threats, follow herds of game, or roam great distances across vast grasslands and forests. As a second line of defense, when we voluntarily fast for a day or so, as insulin levels decline, lipolysis or lipid metabolism occurs, which liberates FFAs, which may be used for ATP generation in place of glucose. And finally, with longer periods of food deprivation, free fatty acids will facilitate ketone formation. Ketones are acids made in the liver that provide an alternative energy source for the brain and heart muscle.

After thirty to forty minutes of cardio exercise, we have seen an improvement in our clients' energy levels, a reduction of inflammatory markers, and better blood glucose levels—the effects of which may last as long as three days. Resistance training designed to improve endurance has well-documented benefits for musculoskeletal health, as well as improvement in cognition—especially in executive function.

MUSCULAR MASTERY

Muscle, a remarkably flexible tapestry of interwoven cells, has been essential to the survival of our human species and a source of our creativity. Michelle Dorrance told us that dance is the physical manifestation of boundless creativity. She said, "The reason that tap dance has the aesthetic or the explosiveness or the articulation that it does is because of the kind of sound that you want to achieve. In order to create a sound with a part of your foot, you have to lift a specific part of your foot, or have both feet briefly hovering above the ground and to stay there."

Our upright-walking hominid ancestors made their appearance on the world's stage 3.5 to 4 million years ago. *Homo sapiens* evolved three hundred thousand years ago, at a time when hunter-gatherers were in competition with large predators.[9] Compared to our spidery brain cells, which consume twenty-two times more energy per unit, myocites or muscle cells are a marvel of efficiency.[10] For 99 percent of our evolutionary history, we have had a highly mobile lifestyle living in small groups. Among surviving hunter-gatherer people like the San of South Africa, the Aché of Paraguay, and the Hadza of northern Tanzania, men and women still average six to nine hours of physical activity per day.[11]

Skeletal muscles, attached to the bones and cartilage, support our body posture and joint stability, which enables us to absorb physical jolts. We also have specialized muscle fibers: slow-twitch (for endurance) and fast-twitch (for explosive movements). Most people have an equal proportion of slow- and fast-twitch muscle fibers.[12] Slow-twitch muscle fibers are smaller in diameter, thrive on oxygen, and are well articulated in marathon runners who remain active for six to eight hours at a time. Champion runners have been shown to have more than 90 percent slow-twitch fibers in key muscles. In contrast, fast-twitch muscle fibers do not rely on oxygen, they contract faster, and produce greater force. As a result of genetics and years of rigorous training, the Jamaican legendary sprinter Usain Bolt and sprinters like him may have 73 to 76 percent fast-twitch muscle fiber.

A pioneer in exercise physiology, the late Duncan MacDougall, professor emeritus at Canada's McMaster University, spent decades scrutinizing the chameleon-like adaptability of skeletal muscle. In his book *The Physiology of Training for High Performance*, MacDougall acknowledged that the process that causes muscles to bulk in resistance training is not fully understood. He postulated that it represents the body's attempt to protect itself from the protein damage that accrues from repeated muscular contractions. This type of exercise improves insulin sensitivity, prevents age-related muscular decline, and adds proteins to muscle fibers.

A recent study showed that a significant increase in strength and endurance can be attained by resistance-trained individuals with just three thirteen-minute weekly sessions over an eight-week period.[13] More weight training leads to more muscle mass. Endurance exercise, on the other hand, causes an increase in cellular mitochondria, muscle cells, and capillary networks.

"PAIN DON'T HURT"

Jake, forty-four, a genial, square-jawed hotel owner, credits his career success to lessons from team sports. He said, "Being on soccer, baseball, and volleyball teams in high school and college helped shape me with leadership skills, a knack for perseverance, and a serious work ethic. It's the kind of training that you may not get elsewhere in the world. It teaches you to cope with mental adversity."

On Jake's first visit to the MetaKura Clinic, he was sweating profusely after a night of heavy drinking. He told us he had made the appointment because he had reached a point where he had begun to take an accounting of his life. His first health-related surprise came at twenty-eight years of age, after he returned from his honeymoon. His cardiologist informed him that his triglyceride level was 768 (normal is below 150 mg/dL) and he had been on statins to treat high triglycerides for the sixteen years that followed. Jake said, "In your youth, you think you are invincible. At first, I dismissed it and thought, oh well, my family genes are against me. After eight years of working at a well-known nightclub in New York City and partying with celebrities, I realized that I need to get my act together."

Clinic Notes

Jake is the youngest of six children of a Polish Catholic family. He reported that both his parents were forty-two years old at the time of his birth. His father's career as an executive with a multinational firm meant that the family moved a great deal. Jake's father had high triglycerides and died of a heart attack at the age of sixty-nine. His mother was diagnosed with depression, type 2 diabetes, and Alzheimer's. His older brother, who was extremely active as the owner of a landscaping company, died in his sleep of a heart attack at sixty-four.

For Jake, as it is for the one in four who have insulin resistance, the mechanism by which skeletal muscle draws in 80 percent of circulating glucose in the blood after a meal is structurally impaired.[14] Between meals, insulin progressively declines to a level that permits the release from lipid stores (lipolysis) of free fatty acids for any energy needs. With higher insulin levels, there is a disruption of communication of the hormone with target cells resulting in higher levels of lipolysis. Jake's lab reports showed his triglyceride level at 975, nine times above the normal range. Over time, mitochondrial function falters, leading to fatigue or symptoms of chronic fatigue; lower levels of resting adenosine triphosphate are produced in skeletal muscle and cells become less efficient at using free fatty acids to create energy. In people like Jake, this process is accelerated, resulting in fat deposits in the muscle and sometimes muscle pain (fibromyalgia).

We urged Jake to resume his athletic activities. Fitness training improves the delivery of blood to the muscles, and it accelerates the pathways of GLUT4 transporters that convey glucose into skeletal and cardiac muscle.[15] Increased glucose in muscles substantially increases feelings of strength and overall energy.

Jake had a fitness assessment that is part of the MetaKura program and was given a customized regimen of aerobic and strength routines to follow five days a week. One of the ways in which exercise improves cardiovascular function is that it stimulates the growth of new capillaries that nourish both resting and active muscle with fresh supplies of oxygen and glucose. Regular fitness training leads to an increased density of mitochondria in the muscle.[16] As a result, the body relies less on consuming carbohydrates and more on using fat stores, which improves a person's endurance capacity.

Jake said that he was very strict in observing the MetaKura meal plan, especially during the first four months. At restaurants, he queried the staff about the ingredients of the sauces being served. He and his wife started reading food labels closely. He said, "None of my cardiologists [that I have seen] over [the past] twenty-two years have ever made a correlation between how my excess circulating insulin triggers the formation of triglycerides when I eat simple carbohydrates. I see it as the key that unlocked everything, because I understand the long view rather than taking a shotgun approach of more statins. No one else had ever articulated the ramifications that if I manage that one piece of my insulin levels, all my blood work issues will get better." By then his triglyceride levels had dropped to 115, within the normal range.

Just as Jake was completing the MetaKura program, he volunteered to help manage a hotel that had converted into a temporary hospital for Covid-19 patients. "I worked for ninety-nine days without a break. There was no sign of relief in the early days. We watched with horror as the charts and graphs climbed upward in the New York area. If I hadn't lost twenty-seven pounds a few months before the pandemic, I would have crashed. We only had time for one meal at around eight o'clock at night. I doubled portions of protein. My favorite quote these days is from the film *Road House*. When the nurse offers a painkiller before she is about to stitch his chest wound, Patrick Swayze says, 'Pain don't hurt.'"

Motor Abilities, Muscles, and Energy Sources[17]

♦ The energy for physical activities may be provided by a combination of glucose and fat energy systems that work together. The proportion of each energy system in play depends on the intensity and duration of the exercise.

♦ During exercise, skeletal muscle oxygen consumption can increase ten to twenty times versus when it is at rest.

♦ The maximum oxygen uptake (VO_2 max) is the greatest amount of oxygen that can be utilized in the most strenuous exercise. A person's capacity is determined primarily by their genes, although aerobic training can help people improve cardiorespiratory fitness. VO_2 max can vary as much as 300 percent from one individual to another.[18]

Physical strength: *maximum energy used in one explosive act: 100-meter race, weight lifting, gymnastics, yoga*

♦ Fast-twitch muscle fibers can generate high levels of power, have fewer mitochondria, and are easily fatigued because they produce more lactic acid. They can contract thirty to fifty times per second.
♦ They depend on energy from anaerobic (oxygen-free) cellular ATP. The quantity of ATP found within cells is only sufficient for a few contractions. Another high-energy compound, phosphocreatine, combines with ATP to provide an immediate source of energy.
♦ With strength training, focus your larger muscles first and then on your smaller muscles to avoid fatigue.

Endurance: *swimming, power walking, cycling*

♦ Long, low-intensity exercises engage the slow-twitch muscle fibers, contract more slowly (ten to fifteen times per second), and rely on aerobic energy.
♦ Slow-twitch muscle fibers are rich in mitochondria and have a greater concentration of aerobic enzymes.

MOVEMENT, YOGA, AND DANCE

For those who shudder at the idea of being in a gym surrounded by sweaty people, we recommend: "Dance!" Increasingly, studies have linked movement with improved cognition and mood regulation. Allegra Fuller Snyder, the former head of the dance department at UCLA, has said, "Dance is more than an art. It is one of the most powerful tools for fusing the split between the two functions of the brain, the fusing of the logical with the intuitive, the fusing of analytical perceptions with sensory perceptions."[19]

Yoga offers similar benefits. Between 500 and 400 BCE, yoga's spiritual roots arose from the Sanskrit sutras (a stitch, a thread, or a teaching that is easy to recall) of Patanjali's classic, *Yoga Sutras.* Hatha yoga *asanas, pranayamas,* and *samyama*—postures, mindful breathing, and meditation—are designed to help individuals achieve a peaceful inner state with self-regulation. According to Patanjali, yoga postures or asanas are used to physically control the body in preparation for controlling the mind. "Every category of asana has a therapeutic purpose," Anahita Sanjana, a respected yoga teacher in India, tells us. "Forward-bending asanas calm the mind; ones where you stand upright help you connect to the earth and feel more grounded; backward bends open the heart and alleviate depression. We believe that the body is a condensed form of each person's patterns of thought."

EXERCISE, GENES, AND VITALITY

The body's ability to use oxygen during aerobic or cardiorespiratory fitness is measured in maximal oxygen uptake (VO_2 max), the metabolic rate. In a number of large-scale studies, the genetic contribution to individual differences in VO_2 max has been found to be around 50 percent.[20] Other genetic factors influencing an athlete's performance include body size, cardiovascular traits, muscle fiber types, and motor coordination.

Fitness Fuel for Improving Athletic Performance

- L-carnitine and coenzyme Q10 supplements (as needed based on lab tests)
- Natural antioxidants like cabbage, broccoli
- Omega-3 and omega-6: salmon, anchovies, flaxseed, walnuts

> ♦ Tryptophan and other essential amino acids: watercress, seaweed, soy protein, egg whites
> ♦ Iron and magnesium: spinach, beans, unsweetened cacao (70 percent)

AGE NO MORE

Age-related loss of muscle mass is called sarcopenia. The associated muscle weakness can lead to frailties and may make older people more susceptible to falls and fractures. Muscle biopsies have shown the decline of muscle size between the ages of twenty years and seventy years and suggest a loss of skeletal muscle of about 0.26–0.56 percent per year.[21] At times, we have found that some patients with marked symptoms of tiredness and not overcome by exercise can be helped by taking L-carnitine, sometimes along with coenzyme Q10 to boost mitochondrial uptake of free fatty acids. Resistance exercise is also highly recommended, as it increases skeletal muscle mass and strength.

Sarcopenia can be delayed to some extent by exercise, as training adds structural proteins and causes cellular changes that can offset the effects of atrophy. Increased exercise can produce greater numbers of cellular mitochondria, increase capillary density, and increase the mass and strength of connective tissue.[22] The effects of age-related atrophy are especially pronounced in people who are sedentary, and the loss of muscle cells can be seen in trouble with locomotion, balance, and posture. Problems with locomotion and balance can also cause various injuries due to falls.

FLORA'S "WOW" MOMENT

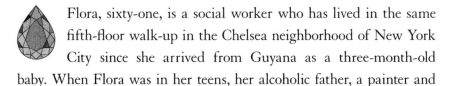

Flora, sixty-one, is a social worker who has lived in the same fifth-floor walk-up in the Chelsea neighborhood of New York City since she arrived from Guyana as a three-month-old baby. When Flora was in her teens, her alcoholic father, a painter and carpenter, left the family home, and her mother began a neighborhood nanny service. When Flora stepped in to help, she found her calling in tutoring and later counseling young children. She came to the clinic after a diagnosis of diabetes.

Her mother also suffered from diabetes. Flora said, "For six years, my mother took her medications, watched her diet, and walked in the neighborhood. As her caregiver, I accompanied her to hospital visits as she developed glaucoma and went into kidney failure. Eventually, I had to sign a form to agree to have her leg amputated. I don't want my children to have to do that."

Flora had a horrifying experience when she was young that ultimately led her to unhealthy eating and weight gain. She told us, "When I was eleven, my mother sent me to a neighborhood store on an errand. A man followed me into our building and almost raped me. That incident stole my teenage years. After that, I only left my home to go to school. And I took to sweets. I gained weight to the extent that when my niece was born just as I finished high school, people thought that I was her mother."

Flora was diagnosed with diabetes when she was fifty-five years old and has managed it with dietary restriction and medication. But her favorite approach to reducing her blood sugar is to run. As she said, "Running helps me feel free, it's just me and the world. It gives me a sense of euphoria and accomplishment. After I finished my third marathon last year, I thought, you might be sixty and overweight, and it may take you seven hours to finish, but look at all the medals you've won. When you run the New York Marathon and begin the race in Staten Island, you see people in wheelchairs, amputees, or blind people all participating in the marathon. It empowers you to keep going."

Clinic Notes

Flora said that her father died of alcoholism in his fifties, as did one of her siblings; her three paternal uncles lived into their nineties, although they had Parkinson's, Alzheimer's, and dementia. Her maternal grandmother and mother had diabetes mellitus, and her mother had a severe episode of depression while in her thirties.

Looking back, Flora thought she might have been dyslexic (not uncommonly seen with insulin resistance) as she struggled at school and still finds writing somewhat challenging. Her childhood meals featured beans and rice every day, with plantain salads and fried food. Flora has been seeing a cardiologist for tachycardia, a very rapid heart rate, and her doctor implanted a pacemaker prior to her last marathon.

Flora experiences a lot of anxiety at work, where a majority of her clients are undocumented workers who live in fear of deportation officers appearing on their doorsteps or taking their children from them.

Unfortunately, Flora has had some setbacks in her exercise routine. Her family dog, whom she took for walks three times a day, died recently. After being isolated for three months as a result of the catastrophic levels of Covid-19 in New York City, she said that there had been incidents of looting and arson in her neighborhood and she felt less safe. She is now working from home and does not leave her apartment for days at a time.

The impact of exercise on her health is clear, because once she withdrew from her normal level of activity, Flora gained sixteen pounds in five months and her blood sugar markers increased (the average blood sugar test showed an increase in HbA1c from 5.5 to 6.7 percent). To get her back on track, we advised her to undertake forty minutes' walking or eight thousand to ten thousand steps daily. This should help to get her glucose levels under control, give a boost to her mood, and potentially help her reduce her weight.[23] Knowing Flora's indomitable spirit as well as we do, we would not be surprised if she decides to run the New York City Marathon in 2021.

Imagine that you were offered a supernatural elixir that increased your life span, made you look younger and more beguiling, fired up your brain synapses until you were brimming with creativity, and showered a confetti of endorphins your way that made you so happy that you wanted to dance. That elixir is exercise.

CHAPTER 9

Enriching Cognition: Thoughts, Mood, and Memory

When people will not weed their own minds, they are apt to be overrun with nettles.

—Horace Walpole, English writer

The human mind is the essence of every emotion you feel, every thought you have, every sensation you experience, every decision you make, every move you make, every word you utter, every memory you recall...in the truest sense it is who you are," wrote Adam Gazzaley and Larry Rosen in their book, *The Distracted Mind*. The brain, endowed with nearly one hundred billion pinkish-gray, tree-like shaped neurons, has been hailed as the most complex object in the universe. Neurons in the brain's cerebral cortex receive as many as ten thousand signals from the synapses of hundreds or thousands of other neurons. But it is not known whether neurons respond to all of these pulses with equal intensity.[1] At its essence, these chemical messengers can excite or suppress a nearby neuron to generate behavioral responses such as feeding and motivation. With only 2 percent of the body's mass, the human brain devours 20 percent of our body's energy, making it especially sensitive to changes in the metabolism.[2] Because the mind regulates the flow of energy and information, when brain signaling is perpetually clouded by chronic elevations of insulin, do changes occur in our perceptions and moods?[3]

As morning snow swirled outside Boston's Massachusetts General Hospital's Center for Biomedical Imaging, forty-two adults, all under the age of fifty, awaited their turn to be strapped into pearl-white functional MRI (fMRI) machines. They had volunteered to have brain scans for a study to investigate the effects of food choices on cognition. A week prior to the study, the volunteers had been divided into three groups; one third had followed their normal diet, the second group did the same but had fasted twelve hours prior to arriving at the hospital, and the third group was placed on a ketogenic meal plan (high fat, moderate protein, low carbohydrate). Once inside the fMRI, subjects were asked to observe a white cross on a black screen and then let their minds wander as the scanner recorded changes in blood flow and brain activity. In the first round of experiments, for those volunteers who had followed a regular diet, the scanner, which was programmed at very high levels of resolution, showed the firing up of neurotransmitter activity of a brain fueled by glucose. In sharp contrast, in those volunteers who had fasted or had observed a ketogenic diet, the neuronal synapses leaped into action one and a half times faster and more regions of the brain lit up. To verify the results of this first-round experiment, all the subjects were then asked to drink identical quantities of liquid forms of glucose and ketones (hydroxybutyrate). Dr. Lilianne Mujica-Parodi, a professor in the Department of Biomedical Engineering at Stony Brook University's Renaissance School of Medicine in New York, who led this series of experiments, told us, "Using ultra-high-field fMRI, we observed unstable communication between brain regions for people on a regular diet—we call this 'brain network instability.' Because insulin resistance starves neurons of glucose, we observe that even over short periods of time, neurons transmit their signals more slowly. Over time, the loss of fuel seems to cause parts of the brain to atrophy. We hypothesize that, as people get older, their brains start to lose the ability to metabolize glucose efficiently, causing neurons to slowly starve. Looking at brain scans, both functionally and structurally, it appears that diabetes accelerates the process of brain aging." The most surprising finding overall in Dr. Mujica-Parodi's series of studies was that brain network stability begins to decline around forty-seven years of age, with the most rapid process of destabilization occurring after the age of sixty years.[4]

The modified MetaKura dietary approach offers the cognitive benefits described in this study, while avoiding the known harmful effects of classic ketogenic diets, such as dehydration, acidosis, and high triglyceride levels, not to mention kidney stones and low blood pressure.

Neurotransmitters and hormones are indispensable messengers to the brain that control a range of bodily functions. As higher levels of the hormone insulin become normalized with insulin resistance, cognitive deficits grow. At our clinic, we see daily evidence, now broadly supported by medical researchers and clinicians, that chronic elevations of insulin affect cognition, mood, and brain plasticity. In this chapter, we will examine the connection between an unbalanced metabolism and the explosive occurrence of autism,[5] anxiety, and Alzheimer's.[6,7,8] We believe the critical link in the rise of these disorders, among other factors, is insulin resistance. Some population-wide studies might have findings that are contrary to our conclusions, but based on thousands of firsthand clinical encounters and a recent rush of scientific publications, we believe that the evidence is decisively moving in our favor.[9] Poor glycemic control as seen with type 2 diabetes is associated with loss of memory, reduced executive control, and slower cognitive processing speed. Scientists and physicians now widely accept that people with diabetes are at a 60 percent greater risk of developing dementia.[10]

MYSTERIOUS MENTAL LAPSES

Charlotte, forty-one, a photojournalist, joined the MetaKura program, she said, as much for her brain as for her body. "I come from a family that doesn't live long. Plus we have a checkered history of mental illness."

Charlotte is the youngest of four siblings. She said her older brother had a narcissistic personality disorder and was an alcoholic. "Eventually, he wore out his body and passed away," she told us. "My older sister was a schizophrenic and suffered from chronic pain. She took OxyContin for twenty-five years and was very deeply addicted. She died recently." Charlotte added, "You could say that I'm a bit crazed with the notion that life is very fragile. Every now and then, I have a sense of nail-biting fear. A year ago, I hit a deer while driving in New Hampshire, and that threw me off for a few weeks. Recently, my partner was hospitalized for severe chest pains."

Although Charlotte has had some experiences that would frighten anyone, we asked her whether her anxiety had ever led to clinical depression.

She told us she hadn't but explained, "For a while, as I kept moving through jobs every two to three years, I also moved through relationships. At times, I was depressed about not finding someone who liked me for the long term." Charlotte smiled. "Fortunately, all that changed in 2005 when I met Frida, my partner."

While Charlotte has no history of mental illness, she has suffered from what she called "scary blackouts." When the first blackout happened, she had been on some antibiotics following dental work.

"The last thing I remember is having my medication with ice cream. When Frida came into the bedroom, I had thrown up and did not know who I was. At the emergency room, I became aware that they were putting me in a CAT scan machine. But I was not conscious of what I was saying and doing. I kept asking for my dog who had died a couple of years earlier. This lasted for four or five hours."

The second, and most severe, occurrence was in 2012. As she told it, "I was invited to meet an academic publisher in New Jersey to discuss a book project. At the restaurant, we had to walk up six flights of steep stairs. When I got to the top, I didn't know what I was doing. However, I knew I had to keep that sensation to myself. I excused myself to go to the ladies' room and called my partner. I said, 'I don't know what I'm doing here.' Throughout the lunch, I could not organize my thoughts. My responses didn't connect. As soon as the meeting ended, I drove myself back to a New York City hospital, where Frida was waiting for me. On the drive back to the city, when I made a pit stop on the freeway, I worried that I wouldn't be able to recognize my car. The hospital did a CAT scan and MRI and didn't find anything. There were other incidents, but they were not quite as unsettling."

Charlotte also expressed some general health and weight concerns. At five foot eight, she said, she had weighed 125 pounds for years. But playing multiple sports led to a knee injury, which subsequently required surgery three years ago. After the surgery, she added forty pounds to her weight and had been worried about it ever since.

Clinic Notes

Charlotte's paternal grandfather had gout, a sign of insulin resistance, and her grandmother, she said, was barrel-shaped. That side of her family "died young." Her father had a paunch and her brother, who had a history of alcoholism, weighed at least three hundred pounds at the end of his life. Her last surviving brother has autism and lives in a nursing home. Charlotte's mother's side of the family is of German descent. She said they were all over six feet tall and appeared thin; however, a few had rounded bellies.

We suggested to Charlotte that her blackouts were caused by a combination of her choice of breakfast, oxygen depletion from climbing stairs, and hypoglycemia or lack of glucose to the brain. Charlotte's tests indicated that she was insulin resistant. Her typically high insulin levels were further elevated when she gulped down instant oatmeal the morning of her New Jersey appointment and ate ice cream after her oral surgery. The simple sugars in these foods exaggerated her panic attacks and caused her to have an impaired executive function response. In order to ameliorate her hypoglycemia, we advised Charlotte on the importance of including proteins with her meals. With episodes of hypoglycemia, cognitive impairment can be induced by consuming foods that quickly break down as sugar in your digestion. Low blood sugar episodes that occur three to five hours after eating sugars may be recurrent for people with insulin resistance.

Charlotte requested that her meal plan be based on the theme of simplicity and farm-fresh food. She said she could easily eat the same thing day after day and did not have to "be blown away by complex flavors." We advised that her diet be modified to contain a rich variety of wholesome vegetables accompanied by proteins. Further, we stressed that she avoid trans fats with simple sugars, such as varieties of nondairy creamers, as these interfere with the brain's synaptic plasticity, or the strength of communication signals between neurons that affect learning and memory. These "glycation end products" accelerate the production of plaques in the brain and are linked to Alzheimer's. They are also responsible for chronic inflammation and, as we saw in Dr. Mujica-Parodi's research, reduced neurotransmitter activity.

To boost her metabolism and brain health, we also urged Charlotte to adopt an exercise routine that she enjoyed. She dismissed gyms and exercise classes as being "of no interest." Instead, she became an avid fan of pickleball, a paddle sport that combines elements of tennis, badminton, and table tennis.

At the conclusion of the six-month program, Charlotte commented, "The MetaKura program has turned on my pilot light. I feel a lightness of being."

CONSCIOUSNESS AND NEURONAL ACTIVITY

Some of our patients who have been prescribed medications for mental health issues have expressed frustration at the need for their doctor to try different combinations before finding something that works. Their experience with us has been much more straightforward. Endocrinology has a very different approach in that we can measure glucose to a billionth of a gram and prescribe treatment approaches accordingly.

According to a recent study from the University of California, Berkeley, depression symptoms can differ significantly among patients, and about half of all people with depression fail to respond to medication.[11]

In close collaboration with their psychiatrists, and if it is safe to do so, we suggest that our patients gradually stop using (or lower the dose of) their antidepressants, especially as a certain type of these drugs called selective serotonin reuptake inhibitors (SSRIs) commonly result in weight gain.

The two disciplines of neurology and psychiatry have long-standing ties. Neuroscientists like Dr. Prisca Bauer from the University Medical Centre Freiburg in Germany believe that unraveling the mysteries of consciousness can create pathways for new therapies for mental illness.[12] People with depression, for example, may feel that others are judging them. Those affected by trauma may be more emotionally closed off. Neuroscience looks at the brain and behavior. A cogent explanation of consciousness remains one of the major unsolved mysteries of neuroscience.[13] One answer was offered by Marvin Minsky, co-founder of the Computer Science and Artificial Intelligence Laboratory at MIT. A posthumous tribute described him as "rigorous, tough-minded, iconoclastic, daring, whimsical."[14] Minsky famously said, "What magic trick makes us intelligent? The trick is that there is no trick. The power of intelligence stems from our vast diversity, not from a single perfect principle." He contended that the human mind is comprised of at least four hundred mini-mind modules, each of which evolved to execute specific tasks. Once integrated, they create a sense of consciousness. As neuronal networks become unstable with progressive insulin resistance, the acuteness of our perception or consciousness is inevitably altered.

In 1921, Dr. Russell Wilder of the Mayo Clinic wrote a paper showing that more than 50 percent of his patients with epilepsy had seen dramatic improvements in lowering the frequency of seizures by following ketogenic or insulin-regulating diets.[15] Today, with some excitement, scientists anticipate breakthroughs using new discoveries of brain proteins and signals, along with metabolism-based interventions, to treat complex neurological conditions like bipolar disorder and Alzheimer's.[16]

COGNITIVE RESILIENCE

For authoritative insights on brain function, we spoke to Barbara Sahakian, professor of neuropsychology at the University of Cambridge, who
has an extensive body of work on cognition. "Problems of mental health
are problems of cognition; you've got differences in how someone thinks,"
she told us. "A person with depression may be more inclined to notice
someone frowning or may be biased to remember sad events over positive ones. A person with schizophrenia may be making the wrong associations leading to psychotic thinking, including delusions and paranoia."
The second important point that Dr. Sahakian makes is that in 2008, she
was invited to be part of a British government initiative initially called
Mental Capital and Happiness. "I told them that happiness is a momentary feeling, like when you fall in love or get a promotion. Instead, mental well-being, which is a more permanent state, should be the goal that
we aspire to." Her point was taken, and the name was changed to "Mental Capital and Wellbeing."

Dr. Sahakian has identified two types of cognition that are essential
for emotional regulation. "Cold cognition involves paying attention,
complex problem-solving, planning, and other aspects of executive function," she explained. "Hot cognition is concerned with social and emotional
intelligence. Intriguingly, the neural networks for these two types of cognition include different areas of the brain. Cold cognition involves brain
networks including areas such as the frontal lobe and the hippocampus. This latter area is associated with memory, whereas hot cognition
involves neural networks that include areas of the limbic system such as
the amygdala, which govern our emotions." Dr. Sahakian explained that
if you have a stressful day, there may be increased activation of the brain's
amygdala. To regulate your emotions, you may need to use your cold
cognition, including "top-down" cognitive control by your frontal cortex,
over your amygdala, to help you think more rationally and not be over-
whelmed by your emotions.

Dr. Sahakian has studied serial entrepreneurs and high-level managers, mostly in their fifties with similar educational backgrounds. "Both groups made high-quality decisions most of the time when we measured their cold cognition. In terms of risk-taking during 'hot' decision-making, the entrepreneurs showed risky betting. The managers were more conservative and did not show the same degree of risky betting while making a hot decision. The entrepreneurs demonstrated higher cognitive flexibility and were able to find adaptive solutions, whereas the managers were less cognitively flexible and got stuck on unsuccessful solutions. The entrepreneurs' risk-taking patterns, associated with hot cognition, were similar to those of seventeen to twenty-seven-year-olds."

In our clinic experience, people with insulin resistance may have challenges with both types of cognition. Most frequently, we see other cognitive challenges, such as patterns of depression and loss of memory. Senior lawyers, financial analysts, or others in professions that demand analysis, problem-solving, and creativity come to our clinic because they are worried that they have lost their mental sharpness. Once the effects of excess insulin are arrested early on the MetaKura program, improved cognition is usually one of the first changes reported by our patients.

A longitudinal national study in Finland tested eight thousand people in 2000 and then followed up with half of them ten years later. Participants were briefly shown ten words and asked to recall them. Insulin resistance was an independent predictor of a decline in verbal fluency.[17] We are of the opinion, and Dr. Sahakian agrees, that the human gift for cognitive resilience should never be underestimated.

Luv Michael

Nine young men smile as they stand shoulder to shoulder in crisp white chef's coats and cobalt blue aprons and baseball caps. They are in the commercial kitchen of Luv Michael, which produces organic, gluten-free, and nut-free products. This nonprofit's award-winning granola is sold in sixty locations and on JetBlue Airlines. Dr. Lisa Liberatore is an accomplished ENT (otolaryngologist) to whom we refer many clinic patients for sleep apnea. She is the co-founder and the vital force behind Luv Michael, which is named for her son who has autism. Luv Michael's mission is to train, educate, and employ people on the autism spectrum.

One day, Lisa brought twenty-two-year-old Michael to the clinic. She wanted to understand the reason for her son's distended belly, although he exercised every day. She also wondered if dietary changes could modify Michael's intense response to situations that he perceived as overwhelming. Following Michael's lab results, Lisa said, "It was an affirmation of the fact Michael's insulin resistance caused the increase in his visceral or abdominal fat. Somehow that knowledge about his metabolism gave me the fortitude to forge ahead. Autism is so complicated that you have to choose where to put your energy."

When questioned about his responses to specific foods, Lisa observed, "If Michael eats gluten, he gets silly and his stomach blows up. If he eats rice, he starts laughing nervously. He cannot focus and starts jumping around. It's like giving him a drug." Our own observations suggest that children with autism tend to gain weight as adults, while their first-degree relatives more often have insulin resistance–related disorders. Lisa said, "Instead of pulling him into our world, my husband and I have learned that Michael needs a world where his food and everything that surrounds him is therapeutic."

In a change that his parents have meticulously planned, Michael and his two roommates have moved into the first model home for autistic adults in Southampton founded by Lisa and her husband, Dimitri, through their nonprofit. This pioneering model combines a home with a faith-based supportive community, which in their case is the Greek Orthodox church located walking distance from the house, and expertise from Stony Brook University.

In her revelatory book *Mind Fixers: Psychiatry's Troubled Search for the Biology of Mental Illness*, Anne Harrington has chronicled the twin pitfalls of approaching mental illness as either a biological condition (the highly contested "chemical imbalance" theory of depression that was promoted by the pharmaceutical industry) or as a crisis of consciousness (a recent editorial in the respected medical journal *Lancet Psychiatry* described schizophrenia "as an unmapped, ill-defined area, perhaps as an iceberg").[18] Because there is a lack of reliable ways for predicting success for treatment, there are high drop-out rates among patients. Many mental health issues make their first appearance during childhood and persist through adult life with complete remission being rare.

Such is the case with general anxiety disorder, globally the most prevalent mental illness, affecting 284 million people.[19] Mignon McLaughlin, the satirical American journalist, wrote, "Love looks forward, hate looks back, anxiety has eyes all over its head." Indeed, as we all know too well from our personal experience, with heightened anxiety, steady waves of thoughts command the emotions, influence belief systems, and penetrate the deepest layers of subconscious thinking. In the landmark Great Smoky Mountains Study that began in 1992, Dr. E. Jane Costello followed nearly fifteen hundred children aged nine to thirteen in the Appalachian Mountain region of North Carolina with anxiety disorder and found the extent to which it lingered throughout adult life. By the age of twenty, 61 percent of the children had at least one diagnosable disorder, most commonly anxiety, and a further 21 percent had subclinical symptoms of stress, bringing the total of those struggling with their mental health to 82 percent.[20]

Signs of an Anxious Personality

♦ Constantly checking the time, news, social media, or other sources of information; poor concentration
♦ Rethinking and ruminating through moments of the day
♦ Isolating oneself
♦ Rigid routines or withdrawal from activity
♦ Physical tics and fidgeting

While the connection between insulin and anxiety is still not fully understood, the hormone plays a number of roles in the central nervous system, including promoting growth and influencing cognitive functions such as memory formation. The part of the brain that is credited with learning and memory retention, as well as neurogenesis, or the creation of new nerve cells, is the hippocampus. This area of the brain is also the location for olfactory memory, or the ability of odors to vividly trigger the evocation of emotional experiences. Scholars have referred to this as "Proustian memory" because of the well-known evocation of dipping madeleine cakes in tea in *Swann's Way*.[21] It helps animals determine if wild berries are safe, as well as when to avoid predatory threats. Similarly, the human brain synthesizes verbal memory and symbolic knowledge in the hippocampus for future decision making.

GIFTED AND DYSLEXIC

Dyslexia is a neurobiological disorder with a genetic origin. Forty percent of affected children exhibit reading deficits within the first few months of formal instruction.[22] Gifted dyslexic children, as shown in a study in Ontario that analyzed cognitive and creative differences in children nine to fourteen years of age, "exhibit strength in expressing humor, problem solving, capturing the essence of an idea, and in synthesizing dissimilar concepts."[23]

Fiona, forty-four, spoke openly of her lifelong difficulty with reading and writing—her likely dyslexia was never diagnosed or treated—yet because she was organized, highly articulate, and easygoing, she was elected president of her class in high school, led her school's all-star cheerleading squad, and was theater director of her school plays. Now a child counselor, Fiona said, "We are now seeing unprecedented levels of anxiety in our children. Social media brings out our primal insecurities and doesn't allow us to work through them. When I was young, if I had an unpleasant interaction, I had a knot in my stomach for an hour, but then I went home and thought about other things. Now, it's different for our children. The phone is with you twenty-four-seven. It starts to become your psyche."

Fiona initially joined the MetaKura program for weight loss, after deciding to focus on her health. As the weeks went by, she grew increasingly drawn to understanding the hidden role of insulin resistance in her life. She saw the insights this mysterious, pervasive underlying condition could offer for the many unanswered questions she had about her family. Her five brothers and three sisters, she told us, also suffered from varying degrees of anxiety. She said, "I had difficulty concentrating. When you are one of nine children, you quickly learn how to get attention. I would put on my tap shoes and be the life of the party. Even though I sensed that I had a learning disability, I was valued by my family and friends for who I was and not how I performed academically. Society now judges my children purely on academic merit. We don't educate the whole person."

Fiona acknowledged that two out of three of her children are being treated for anxiety or learning problems, with one having had to take a leave of absence from school. "Ours is a highly competitive school district, and it's easy for children to feel that they are not good enough. For me, there are three questions I ask myself about my children. Are they keeping up with the things they have to do? Do they seem, in general, to be happy? Do they have friends?"

Fiona attributed her weight gain to her pregnancies and depression following her second pregnancy. She said, "Five years after our wedding, my son was born; I tell him, he gave me the best year of my life, I was a new mom, in a new home. The only problem was that I gained forty-five pounds during my first pregnancy and a hundred pounds while I was pregnant with my twins. I literally don't remember the two years after they were born. At first, I thought it was sleep deprivation. Then I realized that it was postpartum depression. It was as if the lights went off and there was fear lurking in every corner. Everything was flat. I went from being used to a noisy household to not being able to bear to hear a spoon drop."

When we asked her about diet and if she could connect any foods to her behavior or emotions, she told us, "Years ago, every Saturday my husband would bring home hot bagels for breakfast. After eating them, I just wanted to take a nap. I'd feel whipped. The same thing happened when we went out to eat and I had pasta. When I went gluten-free, I couldn't believe how much better I felt. Recently, when I accidentally ate corn, I could immediately feel the effect of food on my brain. That's another thing, I've become very forgetful."

Other health issues that she shared included a bout of shingles one and a half years ago, which she blamed for recurring shafts of pain that run down her leg. She has seen a rheumatologist and an acupuncturist, and the latter offered her some relief.

Clinic Notes

Fiona had dyslexia and was fortunate not to have the debilitating anxiety that affected her children. Most anxiety disorders, including obsessive compulsive disorder, panic disorder, specific phobias, and social anxiety, make their first appearance in childhood and result in overactivity of the right prefrontal cortex.[24]

When Fiona began the MetaKura program, the initial assessment of her diet concluded that her nutritional strengths included a healthy intake of proteins, including eggs and chicken. Fiona had recently acquired an Instant Pot, and she asked to be given a number of recipes to use it on the meal plan that was designed for her.

In its mildest form, the type of forgetfulness that Fiona complained about involves lapses in what is known as episodic memory. Nearly everyone has instances of difficulty recalling information such as where they have parked the car or left their phone or keys. Brain health apps, including some developed by Dr. Barbara Sahakian's lab at the University of Cambridge, have shown positive results in this area.[25] As memory loss progresses, people with insulin resistance may struggle to retain information. Exercise is immensely beneficial in improving cognition.[26]

Contrary to her assumption, Fiona's leg pain was likely not due to shingles. Instead, we told her that it was probably caused by fibromyalgia, a disorder that is characterized by muscle and skeletal pain that is more prevalent in women than in men. We see fibromyalgia as one more feature of insulin resistance.[27] We suspect that when fat is deposited in abnormal sites in the body, it may result in inflammation, which is the body's attempt to remove it. This response is magnified by inflammatory cytokines like IL-6 and TNF-α released by fat cells in muscle.[28]

PLASTIC BRAINS

Perhaps the busiest and certainly the most thought-provoking area of neuroscience is neurogenesis, the growth of neurons, and with it, the idea that our cognitive capabilities are not fixed. Neuroplasticity addresses changes in the brain that occur at a cellular and structural level and is especially significant for the cognitive resilience of the elderly population. In 1793, the Italian *letterato,* or Renaissance man, Michele Vincenzo Malacarne concluded a multiyear experiment. He studied pairs of dogs from the same litter and birds from the same batch of eggs and discovered that those that had been intensively trained had substantially larger cerebellums than those that had not been trained, which led to the question of the effect of training on human brains.[29] A groundbreaking Berkeley neuroscientist, Dr. Marian Diamond, known for her piercing intellect hidden behind a ready smile and, in her later years, her swish of silver hair, created a stir with her studies of rats' brains that showed a stimulating environment of toys and friends changed their brain composition. In 1984, she examined the preserved cerebral tissue of Albert Einstein and found that he had a higher number of glial cells (which support neurons) than the average person. Diamond's work and that of others showed that the brain can grow (or shrink) in two ways. Functional neuroplasticity assesses the frequency and strength of nerve signals or the stability of neuronal activity in the brain's synapses. Structural plasticity looks at the formation of new cells and new neuronal pathways; in other words, the areas of the brain in which neurogenesis occurs or new brain cells are formed. In 2010, Sally and Bennett Shaywitz, co-directors of the Yale Center for Dyslexia and Creativity, used fMRI studies to follow affected children and to show that their brains develop compensatory changes to help overcome their learning disabilities.

Neuroplasticity can also be hard won by challenging life experiences. "By the time I was sixteen, I had been diagnosed with depression," said twenty-one-year-old Ezra when he joined the MetaKura program. "I had racing thoughts, a lot of anxiety, and imagined myself dying. Then, one day in my coursework at college, I read a proverb by Voltaire, 'Perfect is the enemy of good.' That's when I stopped beating myself up. I realized that we try to be perfect, and when we are not, we give up. On the days when I didn't exactly follow my meal plan on the MetaKura program, I stopped wanting to give up on myself. I taught my brain to react positively."

Like diabetes, depression is a complex, many-faceted disorder. Depression is often linked to adverse childhood experiences, including neglect, and anxiety-causing experiences like abuse show heightened activity in the amygdala.[30] It has been shown to affect 40 percent of people with type 2 diabetes.[31] Both conditions are evidenced by higher inflammatory markers or cytokines, including interleukin-6 and tumor necrosis factor. Postmortem brain studies and clinical tests have shown that the corticotropin-releasing hormone, which is activated during stress response, has been found to be elevated in individuals with acute depression and in those who have committed suicide.[32] The challenge of making links between diabetes and depression is that diabetes has specific diagnostic laboratory criteria and depression can be variously diagnosed by personal interview, subjective questionnaire, or self-diagnosis. However, we find that many of our insulin resistant patients have combinations of chronic fatigue, cognitive impairment, and depression, for which they often report improvement by following the MetaKura program.

FORGET-ME-NOT

Dylan, fifty-seven, is a concert pianist who performs internationally. He joined the MetaKura program after visiting his dementia-stricken mother in the hospital, where she asked him, "Remind me, how long have we known each other?" Dylan, who is also a very dear friend, had heard us talk about the National Institutes of Health's multiyear TAME study to prevent Alzheimer's by regulating insulin levels.[33] Unusually tall and affable, he has been known to lie on the floor all night to care for a sick kitten.

Dylan gave us information on his previous diagnoses and health history. He told us, "I now know that I have ADHD and dyslexia, which made school more difficult, but it was only diagnosed a few years ago. I had severe depression in my early twenties, which was completely resolved with two years of psychotherapy. I found it helpful. A couple of years ago, I had career burnout and felt hollowed out. But I've learned to catch myself by exercising and creating relaxation breaks before becoming too depressed."

He also told us that he had knee surgery that was related to his excess weight. He used to run marathons but currently lifts weights, cycles, and uses a rowing machine. His mother's dementia has been of concern for some time. As he told it, "I first noticed it six years ago when we would call her from overseas. She'd keep asking the same questions over and over. Of late, it has become painful to see her. When my sister went to visit her two hours after I left the hospital, my mother would complain that she had not seen me in a long time."

Clinic Notes

Dylan's father had clinical depression, and his sister's bipolar disorder is being treated with lithium. As noted above, Dylan has ADHD, dyslexia, and depression, and his mother had dementia.

When he was in his twenties, he began to be mindful of his food choices and maintained his weight by running ten to twenty miles on weekends. Unfortunately, by the time Dylan entered his fifties, the years of a heavy international concert schedule had taken a toll, and he was noticeably heavier.

For many of our patients, including Dylan, fear of dying causes them less worry and fear than the prospect of Alzheimer's. Dementia is thought to be caused by a combination of health, genetic, and lifestyle factors. We believe that the disorders of hypertension and arteriosclerosis, which are also lifestyle-related diseases, can impair cerebral blood flow, and increasingly underlie dementia in the very elderly. In the United Kingdom, "type 3 diabetes" (a term we do not favor because we see diabetes as a distinct medical complication) has been used to describe Alzheimer's because the association between the two diseases is so strong. In the general population, Alzheimer's disease affects as many as one in every three people over the age of eighty-five. The rate of Alzheimer's doubles every five years after the age of sixty-five. Because women tend to outlive men, more women than men are affected by the disease.

One impressive ten-year study by Dr. Richard H. Tuligenga and colleagues at the Paris Hospital was conducted in people aged fifty-five to sixty-five. It showed that those with type 2 diabetes had a 45 percent faster memory decline, a 29 percent speedier decline in reasoning, and a 24 percent reduction in global cognition compared with matched controls with normal blood sugar levels.[34] They found even greater differences among those with the highest glucose levels. As mentioned previously, our clinic prescribes the insulin-regulating drug metformin. It is currently being used for the NIH TAME study (Target Aging with Metformin) to gather data on its ability to prevent or delay dementia.

Today, after dropping twenty-eight pounds, Dylan looks younger and feels energized. Watching his discipline with diet and exercise over several years, we believe that he will beat the odds and not follow in his late mother's footsteps.

Your brain is sensitive to your choice of food and your emotional and physical well-being. In addition to the suggestions in the following box, if you are not hypoglycemic, you may consider "metabolic switching" or intermittent fasts, as this fosters brain-signaling pathways that promote neuroplasticity and protect brain health.[35]

Champion Your Plastic Brain[36,37]

Activities

♦ High-intensity exercise increases the growth of nerve cells in the hippocampal area of the brain. Older adults who exercise more regularly have increased brain volume compared to ones who do not.

♦ Cognitive challenges like piano lessons, language learning, and acquiring computer programming skills improved attention, control, motor function, visual scanning, and executive functioning.

♦ Form close social and emotional bonds. The brain is highly vulnerable to environmental influences, and among primates, scientists believe social influences are especially significant.[38]

♦ Relaxation rituals and meditation expand gray matter density in human brain stems; music is a multisensorial activity that promotes neuroplasticity.

♦ Get at least seven hours of sleep nightly.

Food

♦ Strawberries and blueberries (polyphenols with powerful anti-inflammatory and anti-oxidant properties)

♦ Nuts and seeds (vitamin E)

♦ Wild-caught salmon, flax seed, walnuts (omega-3 fatty acids are optimal for central nervous system efficiency)

♦ Cocoa (flavonoids are neuroprotective and can enhance mood and cognitive function)

A PHANTOM ILLNESS?

Adverse childhood experiences can lead to a lack of resiliency and vulnerability that continues into later years. In psychiatry, increasingly, greater emphasis is being placed on understanding the developmental and sociocultural factors that cause trauma and can progress to posttraumatic stress disorder.

Lanying, thirty-nine, a Shanghai-born founder of a recycling company, suddenly found it difficult to walk. She came to our clinic on crutches for a second opinion after she received a life-threatening medical diagnosis of amyloidosis. This is a rare and serious disorder where abnormal proteins called amyloids build up in tissues or organs and impair their function. "My tests were not conclusive, and my internist thought you might be able to help me," she said.

As we went over Lanying's early history, two factors stood out. When she was ten years old, she said she would "get the shakes" and feel tremors through her body. Her mother soothed her by giving her little boxes of raisins to eat. There was also a grim family history of abuse. She said, "My father would take his belt to us children. My mother would threaten suicide and have me read her suicide notes. I was always told not to tell anyone about my home life."

She described the circumstances leading up to her seeking medical advice.

"For two weeks, I've had extreme exhaustion. My body felt so heavy that I could barely sit up, let alone walk to the kitchen. I began to work from home, switching between working and sleeping every couple of hours. It feels like I have 'cement feet' and that I'm dragging myself around like a slug."

Clinic Notes

Amyloidosis is difficult to diagnose, as it involves bone marrow tests or tissue or organ biopsies. We decided to rule out a few other possibilities pertaining to her metabolism. Lanying had been seeing a therapist for post-traumatic stress disorder. One of the side effects of PTSD is a pervasive sense of fatigue. She spoke of using visualization to overcome feelings of stress, and one tool she said that worked was to imagine herself in a pink protective bubble where nothing could hurt her.

Lanying's childhood tremors, panic attacks, and use of raisins to soothe her may have been an indication that her glucose levels were dysregulated from a young age. Sure enough, Lanying's blood work confirmed her insulin resistance. Given her level of anxiety, it was especially important to plan a diet that helped her feel in control. Three months later, with her ability to walk now restored, Lanying said, "The change of diet made the biggest difference in recovering my energy. Today I look at food as delicious fuel. It *is* so true that you are what you eat." By eliminating carbohydrates, she said that her memory had improved. She was better able to concentrate and did not have to "play charades" to remember words.

Another factor contributing to her fatigue was that Lanying was experiencing symptoms of premature menopause. For some women whom we have seen at the Clinic, the hormonal imbalances triggered by insulin resistance may precipitate menopausal symptoms. Several of our patients resumed regular menstrual cycles after a long hiatus once their insulin levels were well regulated. This was not the case with Lanying.

She said that the restoration of balance to all of her hormones, including her insulin levels, has been empowering, as it permits her not to be so self-critical. She continued, "Earlier I would get frustrated with myself. It's liberating to know that it wasn't my fault and instead this is a condition of my DNA. Turning forty, I now think I'm doing the halftime show, and the wonderful second half lies ahead."

Insulin has been shown to alter cognition, as well as the speed of brain synaptic activity. One of the busiest frontiers of discovery in metabolism-related research is its close connection to psychiatric disorders. The dysregulation of insulin clearly impacts neuroplasticity, moods, and memory. Intense learning, novel experiences, exercise, and a well-chosen diet contribute decisively to improved cognition and brain integrity.

CHAPTER 10

Stress Responses: On Mental Resilience

In the deserts of the heart
Let the healing fountain start,
In the prison of his days
Teach the free man how to praise.
—W. H. Auden (1939,
in memory of W. B. Yeats)

Late on a Friday autumn evening, Noel was hurriedly clearing the paperwork on his desk as he looked forward to joining Sunita and friends at a midtown New York City restaurant. Among a sheaf of papers, he came across a lab form that had been sent over by a medical colleague for a patient. It required a routine signature by an endocrinologist prior to an exploratory gastric procedure. Reading the patient's medical summary, it became clear that the thirty-eight-year-old woman had tested positive for a rare enzyme (21-hydoxylase) that Noel and his colleagues had identified years ago.[1] Immediately, Noel knew that he had to contact her and let her know that she had a life-threatening condition.

Gayle said that she was told by doctors at National Institutes of Health that she is the longest undiagnosed survivor of Addison's disease. "I wouldn't be here if it wasn't for that timely phone call." Her much-admired career as an investment banker had come to a shuddering halt after she had fainted on three occasions while attending international meetings with government officials and sovereign wealth fund managers. Prior to her diagnosis of Addison's at our clinic, Gayle had undergone nine years of inconclusive tests at a university hospital. Addison's disease is caused by a malfunctioning immune system that damages the adrenal glands, which are located above the kidneys. A life-threatening Addisonian crisis occurs when the impaired adrenal glands are unable to produce sufficient amounts of the stress hormones cortisol and aldosterone.

In her book *The Search for JFK*, Joan Blair recounts that in September 1947, John F. Kennedy, then a member of Congress from Massachusetts, fell ill on a visit to London. His friend Pamela Churchill suggested he see a physician, Sir Daniel Davies. The doctor diagnosed Kennedy with Addison's disease and told Churchill, "That young American friend of yours, he hasn't got a year to live." For several years after Kennedy's return to the United States, the endocrinologist Elmer C. Bartels cared for the then-congressman at the Lahey Clinic.

In this chapter, we will examine the multifaceted sources of stress—biological, social, dietary, and psychological, among others. As we have delineated in previous chapters, people with insulin resistance are more vulnerable to depression, excess weight, and stress-related eating disorders. Fortunately, we have found multiple solutions that our patients have used to reduce and manage stress, no matter the source.

Our patient Gayle and JFK both suffered from the lack of the stress hormone cortisol, which can help the body respond in times of stress or danger. Animals deprived of cortisol due to the removal of their adrenal cortex in experimental studies are prone to death during times of stress. Interestingly, cortisol does not stimulate a stress response in the body; rather, it regulates it. Stress is an important aspect of our Metabolic Matrix because of cortisol's role in decreasing insulin sensitivity and reducing appetite regulation. Episodes of stress in our patients may result in binge eating (and far less commonly, anorexia nervosa). In the sanctity of our clinic's office, our patients of wide-ranging backgrounds unburden themselves of their anxieties. "Very unhappy at work," "difficult family situation," "recently laid off from her job," or "appeal to insurance for denying prescribed medication" are recurrent phrases in our patients' medical charts. To keep up with their intense work schedules, more and more of our patients have felt compelled to surrender the quieter spaces in their lives, the extra hour of sleep, a walk in the park, or a freshly prepared family meal. We are moved by the courage of our patients. Faced with so many odds stacked against them, despite their physical ailments, each day they continue to try and do their best at work and for their families.

More than anyone in the Western world, an articulate, Montreal-based endocrinologist, Hans Selye (1907–1982), was responsible for popularizing the idea of stress. He called it "the wear and tear of the body." Selye supervised forty assistants and (perhaps cruelly) used fifteen thousand lab animals in experiments for several decades before presenting his model of stress, which he called the general adaptive system.[2] Conceptually, it had three phases: the alarm reaction, the stage of resilience, and the stage of exhaustion. Selye famously wrote, "What is this condition that the most different kind of people have in common with animals... what is the nature of stress?"[3] In 1956, he correctly suggested that the body's mechanism for adapting to stress was primarily controlled by hormones and neurons.

During the 1950s, 1960s, and 1970s, the *British Journal of Psychosomatic Research* published increasing numbers of studies that implicated stress in a range of diseases, including cancer, peptic ulcers, tuberculosis, asthma, eczema, and coronary and thyroid disease.[4]

With insulin resistance, cortisol goes a little wild. Studies have shown that people with Cushing's syndrome, with long-term elevations in their cortisol levels, select high-fat foods twice as often as do normal weight subjects.[5] The late Bruce McEwen of Rockefeller University, who led the field of understanding the neural effects of stress for at least thirty years, coined the term "allostatic overload." This concept describes the interplay between chronic social stressors and their biological consequences. Regular allostatic overload responses are linked to cardiovascular disease, asthma, and migraines.

A CHILD'S DISTRESS SIGNALS

 When Vanessa first came to the clinic as a nine-year-old, she had short bangs and a ponytail. She looked around the room distractedly, restlessly moved around, and asked a lot of questions. Vanessa was accompanied by her tired-looking mother, who worked in sales at a jewelry store in Staten Island. Born prematurely at thirty-four weeks, at a weight of three pounds ten ounces, Vanessa had, her mother said, been diagnosed with ADHD at seven years of age. Although this young girl began to walk in her first year, she had delayed speech. She developed pubic hair by the age of six and now showed signs of going into full premature puberty. Vanessa's mother wanted to know how best to help her only child.

Clinic Notes

Vanessa was four feet seven inches tall and weighed 144 pounds, placing her BMI at 33.5, a cause for clinical concern. Her mother had had gestational diabetes, while her father's family had a history of thyroid conditions. Given the mother's medical history, the likelihood of Vanessa having insulin resistance was high and was later confirmed by her blood work.

The average stages of puberty for girls are: *adrenarche* (seven to nine years old; the adrenal glands "awaken" to produce sexual hormones), *thelarche* (eight to eleven years; onset of breast development), growth spurt (eleven to sixteen years), *pubarche* (average twelve years; pubic hair appearance), and *menarche* (ten to fifteen years), when menstruation first occurs. The age of menarche continues to fall due to the increased size of children today. Girls like Vanessa with premature adrenarche are also seen to be less sensitive to insulin.[6] When we closely monitor such children, their first sign of a distressed metabolism is excessive levels of cortisol.

In our own observations, children like Vanessa oversecrete glucocorticoid hormones with the onset of adrenarche. As was the case with her, that may result in pink striae or skin ridges on the shoulders and upper legs. We urge parents not to dismiss these as "stretch marks" of a growing child. These skin marks are an indicator that the child is at high risk for insulin resistance. As their cortisol measurements rise, these children begin to exhibit the first signs of underlying metabolic imbalances (excessive gain in bodily fat, elevated lipid profiles that increase the risk for coronary heart disease in later life, and in some, elevations of blood glucose levels). Over time, the pink striae will fade.

With insulin resistance, isolated measurements of certain hormones may not reflect their actual functional levels. (See Chapter 12: Hormone Imbalances.) Paradoxically, when the cortisol level of people with insulin resistance is measured, it may be found to be normal. This is because their elevated insulin levels suppress the potency of the long-distance carrier protein corticosteroid binding globulin (CBG) that transports 80 to 90 percent of cortisol and cortisone in the blood across all body tissues. The remainder is loosely bound to albumin in the blood or in free form, where it is biologically active. Therefore, if the "free" levels of cortisol are measured in the blood that are not bound to the depressed CBG transporter protein, these levels are invariably found to be high, as was the case with Vanessa. Vanessa's added belly fat awakened her relatively inactive body cortisone to transform itself to the active hormone cortisol.

Because our frolicsome nine-year-old patient was fond of swimming, jumping on her trampoline, dancing, and shooting basketballs at the hoop on her driveway at home, we advised her mother to encourage all her daughter's physical activities. We also recommended that she stop her morning raisin and nut breakfast granola (too much sugar) and make homemade lunches as a substitute for those offered at Vanessa's school. To the delight of her family, even as she grew three inches over the next year, Vanessa lost thirty-one pounds, changing her physical measurements to well within the median percentile for other girls of her age. The following year, she gained another inch but had a brief setback after she began to eat candies at school. When Vanessa regained seven pounds, she began to show early signs of elevated levels of insulin with acanthosis, the skin discoloration in her armpits and neck.

Surrounded by her supportive parents, and her uncle and aunt who are also clinic patients, Vanessa subsequently won the day by permanently changing her diet and arresting her trajectory toward medical complications. We continue to keep a close eye on Vanessa, as a number of girls who share her clinical presentation of insulin resistance and premature puberty go on to develop polycystic ovarian syndrome (PCOS).[7]

CORTISOL'S CHANGEABLE NATURE

The body has two nervous system responses, the parasympathetic nervous system (PNS), which dominates the "rest and digest" functions, and the sympathetic nervous system (SNS), which is activated for the "fight or flight" response. The amygdala, found deep within the brain's temporal lobe, primarily relies upon a team of three first responders, the brain's hypothalamus, its legume-sized pituitary gland, and the adrenal glands. This triple emergency response team, called the hypothalamic-pituitary-adrenal (HPA) axis, deploys, in turn, platoons of hormones to stabilize the equilibrium of the body's interdependent systems. The human body is continually responding to internal and external stressors like a bacterial infection or a work deadline. If the stress is prolonged, intense, or of a chronic nature, it can result in mood disorders and increase cortisol levels, which may accelerate the symptoms of insulin resistance. Male monkeys striving for status in an erratic hierarchical structure, where they have repeated conflicts for dominance with other animals, exhibit increased levels of plaque formations in their arteries, accentuating their risk for heart disease.[8] With higher levels of cortisol, people are likelier to gain weight and feel tired or depressed—symptoms that can accelerate the onset of diabetes. We know that brain plasticity, the ability to generate new neurons and synapses, is undermined by stress, although there is new hope that the neuropsychiatric disorders like post-traumatic stress disorder that arise from these alterations might be reversible.[9]

Among the hormones deployed by the HPA axis response team are a profusion of steroids called glucocorticoids. While the precise action of glucocorticoids is still under scrutiny, they are known to minimize inflammation caused by infection. However, it is also suspected that prolonged exposure to elevated levels of these steroid hormones increases the risk of Alzheimer's and depression.[10] Cortisol, a steroid hormone that is synthesized from cholesterol in the adrenal glands, is the star of the family of glucocorticoids.[11] It is essential for life, because it supports our cardiac and immune capabilities. Corticosteroids pass the blood–brain barrier quite well and can reach the brain cells.

Importantly, cortisol increases the level of glucose in the blood, but due to its constant fluctuations, its presence is notoriously difficult to measure. Cortisol levels are highest in the mornings and ebb to their lowest point in the evenings. To overcome this variability, in 2013, at an aerospace factory in Augsburg, Germany, scientists conducted an ingenious experiment. They selected 1,258 employees to verify the links between expressions of the stress-related hormone cortisol and insulin resistance.[12] Because cortisol levels fluctuate in the blood and urine throughout the day, Dr. Tobias Stalder of Technische Universität Dresden decided to measure cortisol in clippings of the employees' hair, where its levels are more stable. As is common for people with insulin resistance, among the aerospace employees there was a direct correlation between higher blood glucose levels and elevations in their cortisol. By identifying those employees most at risk for metabolism-related imbalances and offering them nutritional and physical fitness programs, the company could reduce healthcare costs and improve employee productivity.

Presently, scientists are finding ways to target the action of the visceral fat-based enzymes that promote the conversion of cortisone to cortisol.

THE A TO Z STRESS BAZAAR

Commenting on the overuse of the word "stress," in 1997, Richard Shweder, a *New York Times* columnist and cultural anthropologist, once observed, "Stress is a word that is as useful as a Visa card and as satisfying as a Coke... That's what makes the expression a noncommittal (and also noncommitable) response."[13] In an age of uncertainty and new forms of biological and data-hacking threats, stress can be triggered by a wide range of situations and experiences: a momentary twinge of unease at being late for an appointment, anxiety when faced with speaking in public, a persistent achy back or other chronic pain, the ongoing upset of a conflicted relationship—stress is often used as a catch-all explanation for a legion of chronic ailments. Stress is identified as the root cause for the wide scope of physical and emotional ailments. As equally wide-ranging are the host of stress management therapies that are applied to reducing stress, ranging from Ayurveda to music and art therapy, Tai Chi to Zen candle massage therapy. One reason that stress is hard to predict and measure is because responses vary based on differences in people's personalities, thought patterns, or memories of earlier trauma. Popular psychology podcasts, articles, and books on this subject have created a variety of stereotypes. They distinguish between stress hawks, whom we are told are proactive and bold, while others, called stress doves, are passive, cautious, and reactive.[14] Or they prognosticate stress responses by gender and assert that men tend to react to stress with a "fight or flight" response, whereas women are more likely to "tend and mend," relying on their social networks for support. Or they identify personality differences early in life. An "orchid child," it is said, has heightened stress reactivity, unlike a "dandelion child," who can thrive and flourish in any environment.

In his book *Full Catastrophe Living,* Jon Kabat-Zinn, emeritus professor of medicine and founder of the Stress Reduction Clinic and the Center for Mindfulness at the University of Massachusetts, one of the more credible authorities in this crowded field, has written of stress: "Any concept that covers such a broad scope of life circumstances as does this particular term is bound to be somewhat complex. Yet, at its heart, the notion of stress is also very simple. It unifies a vast array of human responses into a single concept with which people can strongly identify."[15]

Stress is hardly a modern phenomenon. After he witnessed the

Great Fire of London in 1666, the British parliamentarian Samuel Pepys confessed in his renowned diaries that he was afflicted with recurring images of horror, suffered memory loss, and harbored feelings of estrangement. Pepys was posthumously diagnosed with post-traumatic stress in an article published by the *British Journal of Psychiatry* in 1983.[16] From the onset of the First World War, an acute form of stress occurred on the battlefield, where, sadly, its corrosive presence still lingers.

Stress can claim a robust American ancestry. Curiously, in its earliest popular presentation as neurasthenia, stress only affected the leading families of America, with symptoms such as migraines, fatigue, poor digestion, and depression, all culminating in mental collapse. In 1925, William Sadler referred to "Americanitis" (a term that he borrowed from the psychologist William James) as "a result of the tension, the incessant drive of American life, the excited strain of the American temperament." Fifty years later, two cardiologists and medical researchers, Meyer Friedman and Ray Rosenman, codified the characteristics of "Type A" and "Type B" personalities and incorrectly, according to some physicians, linked the former to elevated levels of cholesterol.[17] Alvin Toffler, the futurist writer, blamed the "roaring pace of change" for splintered families and societal disharmony.

In the present day, national surveys claim that the major stressors for the public as a whole are work, financial insecurity, social discrimination, a lack of access to medical care, and global warming.[18] But people are fighting back. With a proliferation of yoga studios, wearable sleep-monitoring devices, meditation retreats, and other sources of enhancing mindfulness, there is a burgeoning multigenerational global resistance movement to reclaim a sense of calm in a busy, stressful life.

From an evolutionary perspective, fear is protective. Our hardwired biological responses to stress can ensure our survival. When faced with events like life-threatening viral infections, a car accident, or raging neighborhood fires due to global warming, the body's central nervous system carefully coordinates a calibrated response to maintain homeostasis or a stable internal environment in the face of these occurrences.

Some of our high-achieving patients engage in what might be called "good" stress. They set ambitious professional challenges for themselves and thrive on defying the obstacles that they encounter along the way as they achieve their goals.

In the twilight of his career, the idea that stress was good for us was also championed by Professor Bruce McEwen. In one of his final publications, he wrote, "We conceive of biological responses to stress biology not in terms of engendering a negative state, but as a typically positive, adaptive set of mechanisms that enhance survival. As importantly, we have come to appreciate that stress biology is not simply an 'emergency system,' but rather an ongoing process: the body and brain adapt to our daily experiences whether we call them stressful or not."[19]

However, when an individual's predicaments cannot be readily resolved and they experience stress on a near-constant basis, it can lead to prolonged fatigue, disappointment, and worry. "Bad" stress, if unrelieved, can become toxic to the body.

While many people acknowledge that stress is prevalent in today's society, we don't have objective measures of the stressors that weigh on individuals. It is easy to measure biomarkers within the body, but it is much more challenging to measure the outside forces that led to stress in the first place.

In 2014, Gary Miller, professor of environmental health science at Columbia University, asserted that given that nature and nurture interact in ways that change gene behavior, we need precise ways to measure the totality of the dietary, social, behavioral, physical, and environmental factors that shape a person's health and alter their ability to function both cognitively and affectively. He called this cumulative measurement of health-related exposures the exposome. In other words, just as a geneticist can make logical predictions about a person's health from the evidence of mutated genes in their DNA sequence, medical professionals should be able to use the "exposome" as a means of assessing environmental influences to create better models for stress-related disease prediction and management.[20]

A career and life coach, who wished not to be named, consistently sees professionals employed by large corporations who are disillusioned and unhappy. Yet they were golden-handcuffed to their jobs, unable and unwilling to leave because they needed the pay and benefits to support their families. She observed that the prolonged stress of being in an ill-suited position, stuck in work that no longer had meaning, and bearing the brunt of debilitating corporate politics was eviscerating. These clients feel that they have lost their identities, their authenticity, and their power. To add to this unbearable stress, many lost their jobs when their employers reduced workforce (downsized). Those who were able to cope with the loss had a support system of loving family and friends, exercised to stay physically and mentally fit, some had religious faith to anchor them; some found spirituality in meditative practices such as gardening. Others, unfortunately, sought solace in substance abuse.

Stress-Shifting Strategies

Here are some of the rewarding solutions that we and our clients have found to relieve the stress in their daily lives.

Creative: Pottery, crafts, art therapy
Social: Gratitude, kindness, compassion, volunteerism
Problem-solving: Setting attainable goals
Cognition: Meditation, intense learning, poetry reading
Physical activity: Yoga, dance, exercise
Resilience: Positive self-feelings, focusing on one's strengths

EARLY LIFE ADVERSITY AND PLASTICITY

The adaptability of an organism based on adversity and environmental cues, known as developmental plasticity, can be beautifully illustrated by the gaudy commodore butterfly. Native to Africa, it has orange wings in the wet season and camouflages itself from predators in the dry season by changing to a bluish purplish color. White water buttercup, an aquatic plant found in northwest Africa, parts of America, and throughout Europe, has long, tendril-shaped leaves below the water's surface. To enable it to float on water, the plants' leaves become scallop-shaped.[21]

In humans, plasticity is affected by the timing of the period of adversity. Children younger than ten are more at risk for serious cognitive challenges following a brain injury than are adolescents. Low birth weight is a strong predictor of rapid weight gain in later life. (See Chapter 3, Genetic Legacy.)

When Jorge came to the Clinic as a thirteen-year-old, his paternal uncle Paul, a schoolteacher in the Bronx, was concerned that his nephew, whom he had recently brought over from Bogota, Colombia, had stopped growing. Jorge's father had died when the boy was six years old. Paul visited his nephew after Jorge's mother remarried. He found that Jorge, who had once been a delightful, curious child, had shrunk into himself and barely spoke. Paul offered to have his nephew come live with him in New York City.

When children are not in a nurturing environment, as the result of a psychosocial event, they may stop making pituitary growth hormone necessary for their growth. While there may also be a nutritional component to the problem, there is a link between chronic stress, brain function, and the pituitary gland. Six months later, after Jorge and his uncle came to assess his growth hormone treatment at our clinic, they discovered that he had grown three inches. Jorge and his uncle couldn't stop smiling and hugging each other. As a young adult, Jorge became taller than most of the other men in his family.

"P" IS FOR PANIC

 How often do you panic? Is it a passing sensation like a sneeze, or is it like a persistent cough, an unwelcome presence that follows you around? Our patient Emine was twenty-four years of age when she flew from New York City to Miami for the weekend with three girlfriends to celebrate their college graduation. One evening, she and her friends stepped into a Miami nightclub, dressed in metallic and floral minis with flashy earrings. Shafts of turquoise, pink, and purple light flashed patterns of moving dots across their faces. As heavy bass electronic beat thundered, plumes of smoke drifted in their direction from a stage. Hundreds of braided, blow-dried, bald, and bewigged bodies, all tightly packed together, twirled in trance-like rhythms across a gigantic dance floor.

Suddenly, Emine couldn't breathe. Her heart seemed to explode, and she grabbed her friend with shaking hands as if she were drowning. "I need air or I'm going to die," she shouted over the music in a cascade of tears. Her friends quickly guided her to the entrance of the nightclub. The management insisted that the only exit available to them was on the other side of the dance floor. "I thought I would die trying to get out of the place. I felt a tightness in chest, and my throat felt [like] it was closing in on me," Emine said.

The next morning on the plane home, Emine's friends fell asleep as the plane was rolling down the runway in preparation for takeoff. While boarding, the aircraft had seemed too small and overly crowded to Emine. Once the plane door closed, she became anxious and couldn't think logically. Emine said, "I felt that I had been shut inside a small box. I worried that the overhead bins looked too fragile and might crash on our heads. I began to cry. I tried to calm myself by looking at the sleeping faces of my friends and by listening to music."

Panic attacks, named after the goat-legged Greek god Pan, who terrified passersby with his bloodcurdling screams, are thankfully rare for most people. But, as you have read, bouts of anxiety and depression recur in so many of our patients' lives.

A decade later, Emine, who is now a botanist with the Central Park Conservancy, came to the clinic to be treated for thyroid cancer. After routine tests confirmed that she also had insulin resistance, Emine opted to join the MetaKura program. She continues to closely monitor her diet and exercise routines because she says that the regimen helps her feel calmer. Emine is a first-generation American of Turkish-born parents. She said, "I felt that my parents and grandparents were working so hard at their jobs, and since I was a child, it was my job to be a perfect student." This put a big burden on her. She also lacked confidence, particularly about her appearance.

One obvious culprit for low self-esteem is the pervasive stigma associated with excess weight. Growing up, Emine said she was sensitive to the way people looked at her. She felt that she didn't look good in the clothes like the ones that her friends wore and decided from early on that she was fat. She said, "As you get older, it's more that you want to be healthy and wake up with energy. It's less about what people say."

Panic disorders, anxiety neuroses, and neuroticism are encountered with a more than average frequency in patients who have metabolic syndrome, another term for insulin resistance. Chronic stress disorders change the structure of the brain's hippocampus and amygdala.[22]

DOPAMINE-LACED DONUTS

"Comfort foods," richly endowed with sugar, fats, or salt, are hedonic in the sense they are eaten not for nutrition but rather for pleasure. When faced with stressful situations, these types of foods are more likely to be eaten to induce pleasure through the reward centers of the hypothalamus. They give an instant, gratifying, feel-good fix. They do so because they generate the "happy" neurotransmitter serotonin from the intestine and the amino acid tryptophan, which arises in the brain. Chronic stress can also disturb the hypothalamic-pituitary-adrenal pathway by increasing the production of glucocorticoids associated with increased fat accumulation in the visceral abdominal cavity.

Eating disorders are a result of a combination of genetic predispositions, childhood experiences, and social pressures. Binge eaters may be harder to identify than anorexia nervosa, especially if the individual lives alone or engages in secretive behavior. Comfort food can be addictive because it stimulates appetite-signaling hormones like ghrelin and leptin. It also activates arousal and pleasure signals between endo-cannabinoid cells, which in turn are associated with increased food consumption and lower satiety. When a person engages in habitual eating to trigger pleasure, greater quantities of food are needed to stimulate the happy feeling. There is a strong overlap between depression and eating disorders, especially in women. The American Psychiatric Association has reported that lifetime rates of major depression in individuals with eating disorders range between 50 and 75 percent.[23]

On Stigma

In a classic late 1950s study cited by Janet Tomiyama, associate professor of psychology at UCLA, ten- and eleven-year-old children were shown six images of children and asked to rank them in the order of which child they "liked best." The photos included a "normal" weight child, an "overweight" child, a child in a wheelchair, one with crutches and a leg brace, one with a missing hand, and another with a facial disfigurement. According to Tomiyama, across various socioeconomic and ethnic backgrounds in the United States, the overweight child was ranked last.[24,25]

An unpleasant encounter with weight stigma negatively affects cortisol levels, which can reduce glucose sensitivity and add more fat stores. Worse, for an adolescent whose sense of self is as of yet unformed, it can lead to what are called maladaptive coping behaviors such as food bingeing.[26] Interestingly, many of those who self-identified as heavy in surveys were not overweight by BMI standards. Undergraduate women report high rates of body dissatisfaction, with estimates ranging from 82 to 94 percent.[27]

Recently, Kira, thirty-two, an artist manager in the music industry, sent us a text message with a photo of her bare feet standing on a scale. "I wanted to start your morning with good news," she wrote. "This is the first time I have seen a number under two hundred on my scale in the past ten years!!"

In seventh grade, Kira said that after seeing signs of her best friend's bulimia, she decided to speak to her. Her friend grew angry and retaliated by saying that Kira was too fat to be her friend. Kira said that a few days later, still in a state of shock and confusion, she lightly nicked her wrist with a razor. Her parents immediately took her to see a psychiatrist for the self-harming behavior, as well as for anxiety and depression. Kira said, "I'm very blessed to have a strong support system. My parents have loved me unconditionally and given me tough love. Early psychotherapy helped me to realize that lifelong challenges can be overcome if I work at it. Mental health is one of my passion points. Instead of punishing people, we need to understand why they are behaving the way they are."

Clinic Notes

Kira's clinical reports confirmed that her insulin resistance was tied to earlier bouts of eating disorders, anxiety, panic attacks, and depression. She received a tailored MetaKura nutrition program that she said made her appetite easier to manage. In tandem with this, she followed an exercise routine designed by our fitness instructor, which she said made her body feel more energetic and shapelier. Our dietitian closely monitored Kira's food diary on an app. Simultaneously, we conferred with Kira's psychiatrist to minimize weight as a side effect of her medication. Kira also learned to modulate her extremely challenging professional life with short stress-relieving breaks and healthy snacks during her workday and to increase her hours of rest, relaxation, and sleep.

MENTAL RESILIENCE

Much can be surmised about mental health from a landmark study published in *Nature* in 2008 called "The Mental Wealth of Nations," which had been sponsored by the British government.[28] It distinguishes between mental capital (a person's cognitive and emotional resources) and mental well-being (the ability to develop one's creativity and productivity, to maintain strong positive relationships, and to contribute to one's community). In *As You Like It*, Shakespeare wrote, "One man in his time plays many parts." As we consider five stages of human existence from the perspective of mental stress management, there are important points to consider:

Early childhood: Based on the intelligence test scores of identical twins raised in different households, genetic factors account for 50 percent of intelligence.[29] Parental diets, substance abuse, and overall health contribute meaningfully to the infant's prenatal environment. Good parenting skills and a nurturing home environment are vital to help build self-esteem and communication skills early in life. Conversely, early stress exposure and childhood trauma are potent contributors to a child's lack of emotional resilience and social skills.

Childhood: Education and a supportive and competent learning environment early in life are lifelong sources of mental well-being. A number of children who come to our clinic need ongoing support for learning differences. Advances in genetics and neuroimaging are opening new frontiers in identifying and diagnosing learning differences and mental disorders where early intervention has been shown to play a decisive role. Optimism and self-regulation are standout skills for parents to emulate for their children, along with emphasizing emotional resilience in this phase of life.

Adolescence: For many of the children that we see, the hormonal upheavals of puberty combined with metabolism-loading food choices and stress can expedite the onset of insulin resistance. At this stage, it is especially important for a teenager to develop self-worth, cognitive flexibility, and coping skills to avoid peer pressure. Excessive stress patterns can lead to self-isolation, as well as alcohol and drug abuse.

Adulthood: A regular exercise regimen, a nourishing diet, and regular sleep habits, as well as strong social bonds, can help the individual avoid anxiety, depression, and chronic illness.

Senior Adulthood: Older adults who have invested in building cognitive reserves by continuing to learn late in life, who feel financially secure, and who have emotional resilience are likelier to enjoy this phase of their lives more fully. Equally important attributes include being active contributors to one's community and avoiding muscular decline with resistance training.

Your Awakened Self

According to Buddhism, human existence entails stress and suffering (*dukkha*), which can be overcome by training one's mind. Cultivating positive emotions plays a central role in Tibetan Buddhism. People who find a purpose in their existence, who believe that their activities are meaningful and that their lives have a coherent narrative, are more likely to find equanimity. Mindfulness is defined by Jon Kabat-Zinn as "the ability to intentionally pay attention to and maintain nonjudgmental awareness of one's experience (thoughts, feelings, physical sensations) in the present moment."[30] Seasoned meditators have the ability to generate mental states that are focused, calm, and lasting.

We spoke to an esteemed teacher, the British-born Karma Yeshe Rabgye, whose wisdom we turn to in our own moments of stress. Lama Yeshe practices in the Kagyu tradition of Tibetan Buddhism and teaches at the Bodhicitta and Prajna meditation centers in Chandigarh, India. He said, "Mindfulness meditation (*dhyaan,* or a deeper concentration of the mind) improves a person's emotional balance and flexibility. It helps to reverse the causes of fear and anxiety. The goal of a mindfulness-based practice is to improve one's self-monitoring, to become an observer of one's mind. We encourage individuals troubled by stress and anxiety to use compassion to reappraise the source of their problem."

Lama Yeshe adds, "As the Buddha said in the *Dhammapada*, 'Fear arises because of craving (*tanhā*). For the person who is wholly free from craving there is no grief or fear.' In that sense, with positive reappraisal of problems and by detaching oneself from automatic negative thought patterns, mindfulness offers us a strategy for emotional regulation. In my experience of over forty years, the practice of self-kindness (*bhāvanā*) that accompanies mindfulness meditation helps to alleviate symptoms of stress, depression, and anxiety."

Matthieu Ricard, a French-born Buddhist monk and writer, cites an experiment suggested to the neuroscientist Richard Davidson by His Holiness the Dalai Lama. After examining fMRIs of twenty people who had each devoted ten thousand to fifty thousand hours to meditation, Davidson concluded that "the brain is capable of being trained and physically modified in ways few people can imagine."[31]

Venturing far from the Anglo-Saxon world lie timeless treasures and stratagems in cognitive restructuring. Between 500 and 200 BCE, the Indian sage Patanjali presented the goal of yoga (*chitta vritti nirodha*) as "the easing of mental fluctuations." Practitioners of the ancient Chinese mind-body practices of *qigong* believe that a person's *qi* (vital energy) cannot flow smoothly if there are stresses or disturbances with *yi* (thought or intention). In the respected Ngoma practices of Central and South Africa, across generations, small groups of people have gathered with a spiritual leader to use the rhythms of music and dance to heal their bodies and minds.

Finally, if we think of nutrition and exercise as the conjoined twins of the metabolism, stress-related behavior is the umbilical cord that links them. Given that stress is unavoidable, each of us, with our own chosen path, can devise a positive trajectory for our lives despite the atmospheric turbulence that appears every now and then. There is reason for hope that as we learn more about the stress pathway that influences brain plasticity, neural circuits can be rewired with positive experiences to enable us when faced with anxiety to be more resilient.

CHAPTER 11

Sleep: Circadian Rhythm and Blues

All I know is that so long as I am asleep, I am rid of all fears and hopes and toils and glory, and long live the man who invented sleep, the cloak that covers all human thirst.

—Miguel de Cervantes Saavedra

To Whom It May Concern,

My patient, Sergio Gonzales, is employed by the New York Fire Department, Ladder 39 in the Bronx. In response to a recent request that he change to a night shift, as his doctor since 2015, I must urge your management to reconsider this change in his shift duty. Such a change in schedule would be seriously harmful to his health, due to his preexisting medical conditions.

Best regards,

Noel K. Maclaren, MD

The MetaKura Clinic routinely sends out letters like this for our patients with complications of insulin irregularities who are compelled to do shift work at their jobs in law enforcement, construction, the hospitality industry, or mass transit. For these essential workers, the lifeblood of our cities, especially those who have compromised health, protecting their need for sleep at night can make a difference in their health and longevity. Along with nutrition and exercise, sleep has an all-pervasive influence on our health, our emotions, analytical and reasoning skills, creativity, and fine motor skills. However, although sleep is so essential, it is elusive for so many.

At the MetaKura Clinic, we are often alarmed at the number of New Yorkers who are muddled sleepers, who report chronic wakefulness or otherwise shortchange their hours of slumber. A disharmonious loop ensues; poor sleep makes appetite signals go haywire and triggers weight gain, crippling chronic fatigue, and then quickly slides into chronic diseases. The extra body weight, more often than not, results in breathing arrhythmia or sleep apnea and contributes to chronic disordered sleep. In this chapter, we will explore sleep through the bleary eyes of our sleep-deprived patients. We will dissect the anatomy of natural sleep, the internal chaos that arises between bodily messengers when sleep is interrupted, as well as the emerging associations between compromised sleep, insulin resistance, longevity, and mental acuity.

Evolutionary anthropologists like Charles Nunn and his colleagues at Duke University believe that, compared to other primates that may average fifteen hours of sleep in a day, human patterns of seven hours are skimpy at best.[1] This shortfall, they theorize, began when human ancestors descended from the trees to sleep on the ground, and individuals likely had to spend more time awake to guard against predator attacks. In addition, humans, being the ever-curious busybodies that they are, may prefer making social connections at the expense of their sleep. After all, to a certain extent, going to sleep is voluntary. As their hours of nighttime rest declined, compared to other mammals, humans evolved to spend the largest proportion of their sleep time in rapid eye movement (REM) sleep. This phase of sleep is associated with learning and memory. While it seems to be a relatively simple behavior, it is not only a state of rest or immobility. For example, once Arctic ground squirrels complete their period of hibernation when their body temperature is greatly lowered, they fall asleep, indicating that sleep has distinct functions that are separate from the energy-conserving rest state of hibernation.[2] In humans, military recruits in training averaged 3.2 hours of sleep per twenty-four hours; their instructors noted "droning" behavior, where the recruits were unresponsive or unable to process information. Sleep deprivation is linked to hand trembling, slurred speech, and greater sensitivity to pain.[3]

CIRCADIAN CYCLES IN DISARRAY

This ancient proverb is attributed to Heraclitus, the Greek philosopher: "Even a soul submerged in sleep is hard at work and helps make something of the world." If as we said in the Introduction, the First Commandment of Biology is the concept of homeostasis—where an organism's biological functions are steadied to remain nearly constant over time,[4] the Second Commandment is circadian regulation, or the ability of life-forms to optimize their biological activity at the proper time of day.[5] Indeed, sleep takes up a third of our life, and its absence for thirty-six hours can lead to hallucinations. During slumber, a number of physiological transformations occur; the brain is cleaned of waste materials such as remnant neurotransmitters and myelin by action of the glial cells.[6]

The connection between sleep and memory consolidation is not fully understood. It appears that non–rapid eye movement sleep (NREM) helps to consolidate spatial and episodic memory of daily events. The rapid eye movement phase that follows is more beneficial for procedural and emotional memory integration.[7] During sleep, energy expenditure is obviously conserved and declines by as much as 10 percent. There is also a daily or diurnal secretion of certain hormones such as growth hormone, which may be involved in bodily tissue repairs like muscle or tendons.

Sleep deprivation has been shown to impair the numbers and functions of natural killer T (NKT) cells, which are important in the defense against infections by viruses and bacteria. The consensus on the ideal amount of sleep needed for adults is seven to nine hours. Requirements change over the course of life: as much as 16 to 18 hours in newborns,

10 hours in children, 8.5 to 9.25 hours in teenagers, and 6.5 to 7 hours in the elderly. Sleep disorders are unfortunately more common as we age. For some of us, as D. H. Lawrence said in *The Fox*, sleep is as evasive as "a shadow within the shadow."[8]

CONFESSIONS OF AN INSOMNIAC

Phyllis, seventy-seven, had one of the more unusual sleep patterns that we have encountered.

"I break up my day into eight-hour cycles of activity and rest. They used to last twelve hours, but they are getting shorter since I've been self-isolating [due to the Covid pandemic]. Because I live alone now, I start my day at noon, though sometimes later," she said.

She has a long-standing history of insomnia. "I was told by my mom that when I was just two years old, she would hear a noise at three or four a.m. and come to the bedroom that I shared with my sister. I would be standing upright, holding the crib rail, moving back and forth, and calmly talking to myself. Later, as a student, I could stay up all night without any caffeine. I could get by on a couple of hours' sleep during the week and then sleep for twelve hours straight on weekends."

The "makeup" sleep did not have the desired effect for Phyllis's ability to function the next morning. "In college, I remember having to take an early-morning exam for a required course. I showed up late with no notepaper or a pen. There were three blanks to fill out on a question and my brain wasn't awake. It was horrible! I have never felt so inadequate."

Phyllis related that when her children were young, she coped (barely) with their need to be up early in the morning. "My husband liked to go to bed early, so I would join him. After he fell asleep, I'd stay up until one a.m. or later. I would wake up at six a.m. to make breakfast for him, then go back to sleep and wake up again to take my kids to school. I was always tired. I never remember jumping out of bed and thinking that I was looking forward to another day."

While she did not look forward to starting another day, she was always eager to partake of snacks and had food cravings for sweets. "I'm a sugar freak; the very idea of desserts, cookies, or other treats would help me find the energy to start my day. Now that I'm older, it's not so powerful a need. I can have three cookies and don't need to finish the whole box."

Phyllis has worn a breathing mask to bed for sleep apnea (interrupted breathing during sleep) for two years but has trouble keeping the mask on at night.

Obstructed Sleep

Sleep apnea is a potentially serious sleep disorder where breathing is interrupted frequently during the night. It affects men more often than women in an eight to one ratio. For such individuals, we highly recommend that they are tested and professionally fitted with a mask like a continuous positive airway pressure (CPAP) device.

♦ Sleep apnea is thought to be due to fat deposits around the neck and pharynx, which lead to obstructed breathing, as well as laxity of the soft palate or uvula at the back of the throat, which can be seen when yawning.

♦ Three of every four adults with type 2 diabetes have obstructive sleep apnea (OSA). Sleep apnea is intermittent cessation of breathing resulting in oxygenation impairments (intermittent hypoxia) and wakefulness.

♦ As many as 70 percent of adults and 40 percent of children with sleep apnea are overweight. Importantly, by following the MetaKura program, we have seen patients fully cured of this problem when they achieve targeted weight loss.

♦ In a published study of seventy thousand women followed for sixteen years, those who slept for five hours per night were 32 percent more likely to gain thirty-three pounds or more than women who slept at least seven hours per night.[9]

♦ Ear, nose, and throat doctors may identify someone with OSA to have a deviated nasal septum as a predisposing cause and correct it with surgery.

Phyllis was often tired and told us that she has fallen asleep while driving, and for that reason has avoided making long car trips for the past twenty years. Phyllis had a rather sophisticated understanding of the potential source of her sleep problems.

"For decades, I've believed that my hypothalamus in my brain is broken. It controls my inner clock, appetite, temperature, libido, and physiological cycles. Isn't sleep a physiological cycle?"

Clinic Notes

Phyllis does not have a "broken" hypothalamus, but she does have a series of complications associated with that area of the brain. She also has a family history that points strongly at insulin issues. She has a maternal aunt with diabetes. She described her mother as "heavy" and her father as "a potato." Of the latter, she said he was probably a hundred pounds overweight, although he had periods when he lost weight. Phyllis has a sister, who did not share these weight problems. She believes both her son and daughter have inherited her genes for insulin resistance.

Phyllis has struggled with her weight throughout her life. At age twelve, she was taken by her parents to a weight-loss program. In her forties, she was at her heaviest weight of 328 pounds. Currently she is 224 pounds. We praised her for her weight loss of 104 pounds, which occurred over a two-year period. Because Phyllis has type 2 diabetes, it was imperative that her insulin injections were taken at specific times to avoid life-threatening complications, so we had to stabilize her sleep cycles.

Phyllis has had some academic and emotional struggles. As a child, she was considered a math prodigy, although she also had difficulty reading, which she was able to hide from parents and educators. At the University of Michigan, she was encouraged to study engineering, a subject that did not interest her as much as computer programming. After twelve years of psychotherapy, Phyllis said she still has low self-esteem. She is currently on antidepressants.

Erratic sleep was at the core of Phyllis's problems. We advised Phyllis on some commonsense approaches to improving sleep: follow regular relaxing rituals such as listening to music, reading, or crochet an hour before bedtime; exercise as vigorously during the day as her health would permit; and avoid any stimulants, including alcohol, three hours before bedtime.

While we cannot report that Phyllis has fully reformed her nocturnal habits, she has brought more order to her sleep cycles than ever before, allowing her to be confident that her insulin doses are well-timed.

ANATOMY OF SLEEP

Sleep and dreaming are closely associated, and dreams can be a rich source of creativity. Samuel Taylor Coleridge wrote of insomnia as "the night's dismay, saddened and stunned the coming day."[10] Dreams, according to the Maori people of New Zealand, were believed to arise from one's spirit (*wairua*) leaving the body and wandering about. Whether they delivered ill omens or prophecies of good fortune, dreams were seldom ignored. Without sleep, you cannot dream, and a coordinated series of physiological occurrences are required for sleep to occur.

Sleep Onset: Nearly two hours before sleep, the small pineal gland at the base of the brain begins to dispatch its emissary, the hormone melatonin, which induces feelings of relaxation and sleepiness. Mysteries continue to swirl around this hormone, although it has proved useful in countering jet lag.[11] Melatonin has been shown to have influence on GABA (gamma aminobutyric acid) neurotransmitters, which inhibit or calm brain activity.[12] Another role of the pineal gland seems to be to arrest the onset of puberty. When a rare tumor such as pinealoma impairs the gland in young children, premature puberty can result, especially in boys. It has also been shown that girls who have total vision loss also experience premature puberty, possibly because they cannot perceive daylight and generate melatonin normally. The pineal gland of birds and mammals is influenced by the light in their immediate surroundings. When sleep is disrupted, as it was for Phyllis, the pineal gland can reduce its melatonin production, kicking off a cycle that results in more interrupted sleep.

In addition to melatonin, a chemical called adenosine triphosphate (ATP) contributes to sleep preparation. During the day, ATP molecules busily transfer energy to cells for life-giving processes like muscle contractions. By dusk, there is a buildup of adenosine levels in the central nervous system. A steady elevation of adenosine molecules also promotes sleepiness.

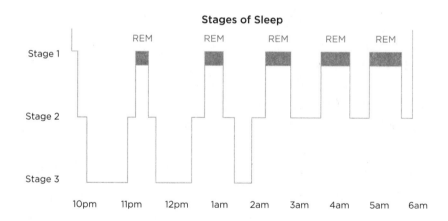

Patterns of Sleep: Based upon studies using electroencephalograms (EEGs) of the brain, sleep is divided into stage 1, stage 2, stage 3, and REM, each of which lasts between sixty and ninety minutes. Each stage has distinct brain waves and physical features. The first phase, immediately after the onset of sleep, quickly proceeds to stage 2 when the body temperature drops, muscles relax, and breathing slows. Stage

3 is associated with synchronized slow delta waves in the brain, considered to be the most restorative stage, and is associated with growth hormone secretion. This stage is followed by REM sleep, when the brain waves show activity associated with dreaming. The brain wave activity is similar to that seen during wakefulness, but REM induces muscle paralysis, so the body does not move or respond to what is happening in dreams. These sleep phases cycle during the night approximately four to six times, while REM sleep periods increase in number and duration toward the morning. For a person like Phyllis, with unsettled sleep patterns, the completion of only one or two cycles could result in a period of wakefulness.

Sleep coincides with the appearance of a parliament of proverbial night owls better known as hormones. It should be noted that in men, the brain's pituitary gland secretes luteinizing hormone (LH), which in turn stimulates the testes to produce testosterone during REM sleep.[13] Depending on the level of testosterone secreted, it may induce a morning erection (nocturnal erectile tumescence), especially after a good night's sleep. In all people, growth hormone released in stage 3 of sleep enhances metabolic responses, including fat burning, bone growth, and bodily cell repair. Several studies have demonstrated that appetite signals are disrupted following fewer than six hours of sleep. The satiety hormone leptin drops to a low level, while the hunger-inducing messenger ghrelin is elevated to a point where our patients say they wake up "hangry" if they have not had adequate amounts of sleep. Quinn, forty-two, a microbiologist, said, "If I wake up before my usual time, say to catch a flight or for an early-morning meeting, I have this angry, screaming hunger. It's very specific. On my normal routine, I only have coffee in the morning and don't eat until lunchtime."

These nocturnal disruptions predispose the body to weight gain. Rarely, as was the case with our patient Isabel, a strange type of muscular paralysis associated with REM sleep may linger after one awakens.

Isabel said, "The first time it happened, I thought it was a dream and tried to go back to sleep. I awoke and couldn't move the entire right side of my body. I couldn't walk or hold anything. This inability to move after awakening has now happened to me four times. It lasts about ten minutes. At first, a team of doctors admitted me to the hospital and tested me for a stroke. But they couldn't find any proof of that. My theory is that it's caused by stress." Isabel has regular sleep habits, but for many of our patients like Phyllis, their internal clocks need a reset.

TICK TOCK, CIRCADIAN CLOCK

Beginning with the mimosa plant experiment discussed in Chapter 1, scientists set out on a journey to answer the timeless question, what makes us tick? This area of scientific discovery also sheds light on the extraordinary leaps of human imagination. Much admired in the court of Louis XV, de Mairan observed that mimosa plants unfurl their leaves in sunlight and curl them up at night. Even when placed in a darkened space for several days, the plants continued to follow this pattern. He surmised that the plants were controlled by an internal clock mechanism. In 1959, Romanian-born American scientist Franz Halberg coined the term *circadian*. He showed that the pulsating internal rhythms of living organisms are subject to the control of external synchronizers such as the degree of light exposure.[14] In 2017, Jeffrey C. Hall, Michael Rosbash, and Michael W. Young were awarded the Nobel Prize in Physiology or Medicine for their discovery of the molecular mechanisms that control human circadian rhythms. At first, working with fruit flies, they identified clock genes that they dubbed with the immortal names of "period" and "timeless." This trio of American scientists went on to augment these discoveries with another elegant series of findings—regulatory proteins that ebbed and flowed in twenty-four-hour cycles to control the activities of clock genes.

With a high degree of mathematical precision, the central circadian clock in the brain's suprachiasmatic nucleus (located in the hypothalamus region at the base of the brain, which responds to light signals from the eyes to regulate the circadian clock) stimulates food intake, energy expenditure, and daily rhythms of glucose metabolism. It processes cues from other independent clocks, the peripheral clock in the gut that controls glucose absorption, while others in muscle, fat tissue, and the liver measure local insulin sensitivity. All of these chimes echo in the chambers of the peripheral clock in the pancreas, the site of insulin secretion.

Phyllis's sleep pattern is an example of what happens when dichotomies occur between daytime light-dark cycles and circadian rhythms—it causes biological pandemonium called desynchrony. A lack of coordination among these clocks, whether because of genetic, social, or environmental reasons, is being studied as a cause of insulin resistance.

Life on Earth is adapted to the rotation of our planet. However, the period of our internal bodily circadian timing system does not match the exact twenty-four-hour rhythm of the outside world and, therefore, must be reset every day. The suprachiasmatic nucleus (SCN) located in the hypothalamus has circadian cells and helps us to adapt to seasonal variations in daylight.[15] A significant contributing factor, or "zeitgeber" (a German word that means "time giver"), in determining the pattern of these rhythms is external light, but also temperature, exercise, meals, and social interactions. Humans appear to have peak performance in their biological processes from approximately six a.m. until noon. Because glycemic control is better during this time period, it would seem preferable for food intake, which is why we strongly recommend breakfast to our patients. In our experience, and that of others, improving the coordination between mealtimes, diet choices, and sleep cycles is a valuable approach to prevent or treat insulin resistance and type 2 diabetes.[16] Prior to adopting the MetaKura diet, Patrick, forty-three, had to shut down in the middle of the day. Patrick said, "At one time, especially because of my food choices, I had to take a nap for one or two hours several times a week. We had company recently, and my wife made a chocolate layered cake. I had a substantial piece and it was like a tranquilizer: I fell asleep for an hour after I ate."

Two Chronotype Profiles

Ted, twenty-eight, works in the patent licensing office of an elite university, although he had once dreamed of having a career as a musician. Lean and muscular, Ted's shorter than average height is made less noticeable by his engaging personality and cheeky humor. Most mornings, stirred by his morning alarm, Ted drains a couple of mugs of coffee and rushes to work from his home in Brooklyn. He doesn't feel hungry in the morning. Ted saves his most demanding projects for the late morning after he has cleared his desk. He cross-trains at a gym most evenings and enjoys winding down at night by watching the late shows with his girlfriend, Mandy. On weekends, Ted and Mandy go to friends' parties or to concerts. Having the freedom to stay up late makes them feel alive.

Jerry, twenty-seven, is head of sales for a small digital marketing agency in Manhattan. He is an enthusiastic cyclist and, weather permitting, can be seen with his friends most days of the year riding across the George Washington Bridge at dawn. At work, his colleagues marvel at Jerry's concentration as he whips though piles of work. By six p.m., however, Jerry begins to lose momentum and heads home for an early dinner. He is usually in bed by ten p.m.

Ted and Jerry represent the "morning and evening" chronotypes or differences in sleep-wake patterns. In a recent study in Saudi Arabia of 540 males and 219 females with an age range of eighteen to thirty-two years, 138 (18.2 percent) were "morning-types," 417 (54.9 percent) were "neither-types" and 204 (26.9 percent) were "evening-types."[17] These chronotype patterns change as one ages. Although culturally and socially we may not-so-secretly envy those who clamber into bed at six a.m. on weekends after a raucous night of barhopping over and over, the data points to the fact that delayed sleep brings a hornet's nest of health complications, including a lower sex drive and impaired immunity. This inverted pattern of rest can be especially harmful for shift workers, who represent 15 percent of the American working population.

After Midnight

Delayed sleep causes bodily disruptions.

- The more growth hormone released in stage 3 of sleep, the more restorative the sleep. Delaying sleep after midnight suppresses the largest GH pulse.[18]
- When healthy individuals are kept awake during the night, bright light causes increased levels of glucose in blood plasma.[19]
- High cortisol levels occur around five or six a.m. to prepare the body for a new day. If the individual chooses to sleep in, they may experience higher levels of blood sugar, heart rate, and blood pressure while at rest.
- Late sleep was associated with a greater increase in fat cells in children as young as two to six years of age.[20]
- Waking up during REM sleep is more likely to make you feel tired throughout the day.

"A Quiet Mind Cureth All"

In his classic work *Anatomy of Melancholy*, first published in 1628, Robert Burton remarked that ancient Greek physicians were well aware of the fact that depressed individuals complained of difficulties falling asleep, maintaining sleep, or of waking up too early in the morning. A recent study by Juan Manuel Antunez, a psychologist at the University of Málaga in Spain, contrasted behavioral patterns between morning and evening chronotypes. Admittedly, the sample size was small, fewer than 2,500 people. He told us that the study did, however, find that morning-type participants had better emotional regulation, highlighting "the assumption of the morning-type as a protective factor against the development of psychological issues as well as the consideration of the evening-type as a risk factor for the development of diverse problems like depression, anxiety and substance use."[21] If you are an evening type, you may heartily disagree with this conclusion. Most of our patients on the MetaKura program with insulin resistance *are* evening chronotypes, and together with their weight struggles, they commonly have varying degrees of anxiety, depression, and sleep apnea. Chronotypes can change. Sunita, who once had a whirring brain at two a.m., now delights in an early-morning fitness routine.

There is likely a relationship between sleep, insomnia, and the regulation of emotion. Experimental data suggest that people with insomnia report more negative emotions close to sleep time as compared to good sleepers.[22] Among the personality traits linked to insomnia are perfectionism, sensitivity to anxiety symptoms, and the tendency to internalize problems. The renowned psychiatrists John W. Winkelman of Harvard Medical School and Luis de Lecea of Stanford have boldly observed, "not only is sleep disturbance a phenotypic feature of many neuropsychiatric illnesses, but it may in fact predispose, contribute to, and dare we say it, cause them."[23]

A STOLEN IDENTITY

Yasmine, forty-nine, called the MetaKura Clinic one morning and pleaded to be seen urgently. Her black hair has a Susan Sontag streak of white. Her slender frame, reminiscent of a dorcas gazelle, is wrapped in a sandy tunic. There is no hint of makeup. She speaks in flat tones about her life and daily routine.

"For the past three years, it feels as if a nasty hacker stole my body. It's as if this cunning thief knew which parts of myself I most enjoy and ran away with them. From having been a chic woman with a Parisian aesthetic, I now tiptoe past my racks of clothes, shoes, and jewelry as if they belonged to someone else." This behavior was in contrast to her usual routine that involved getting up early and having a sparkling home by nine a.m. She says of her home and bedroom, "It was always kept as neat as a shop window. No shoes or food were allowed. Now, if a cup or plate of food is brought in, it stays there *for days*. All I want to do is sleep. It embarrasses me that I am in bed when my husband leaves in the morning and still there when he returns at the end of the day."

She recounted that her husband blamed her change of behavior on the stress of dealing with her older son who went through a defiant teenage phase. In terms of her own health, she went through menopause at forty-two and suffered from jaundice at the age of eight. More recently, she said, "After three years of seeing doctors, I tried to narrow down the causes of my illness to rheumatoid arthritis or fibromyalgia, though neither of them seemed right. Now it's unbearable and that's why I *had* to see you today. My ears hum. My body aches with muscle cramps. I drink Red Bull, but it doesn't help."

The dysregulation of her sleep cycles led us to ask about the possibility of hyperactive thyroid problems. In Yasmine's family there was a long line of women who suffered from thyroid issues, including her sister, who had a goiter the size of a grape. Although we needed to do some tests, her family history and current systems led us to believe that Yasmine had thyroid dysfunction, which is strongly familial.

Clinic Notes

In Yasmine's family, there were many members with enlarged thyroid glands or goiters. Autoimmune thyroid disease is a genetic disorder and is more commonly found in women as compared to men. Women are up to eight times more likely than men to experience hyperthyroidism. Thyroid disease can induce hyperthyroidism (overactive) and hypothyroidism (underactive), as well as a multiplex of autoimmune challenges.* It is well established in clinical practice that hyperthyroidism is associated with insomnia. Because thyroid hormones regulate the speed of all bodily cells, especially with respect to body temperature, Yasmine suffered "hot flashes," which she mistakenly attributed to menopause. Significantly, the increased speeds of bodily functions led to her

---

* Dr. Maclaren refers to these as autoimmune polyglandular syndrome type-2 (APS-2).

weight loss and the principal symptom of fatigue. As with other cases of hyperthyroidism, extreme fatigue, a rapidity of divergent thoughts, and jumping from one subject to another with a loss of sustained concentration can be observed in her case. Yasmine said that she woke up four or five times a night. Her rapid heartbeat, even when resting, contributed to her insomnia.

Initially, we advised Yasmine to stop any strenuous exercise and to consume lots of fluids earlier in the day to compensate for the loss of water from the body through excessive urination. When her blood work confirmed our initial diagnosis, medication was prescribed to slow her heart rate and to regulate her thyroid function. In six months, Yasmine was able to return to living her life the way she wanted.

For some, lacking the powers of Hypnos, the god of forty winks in Greek mythology, sleep may be an evasive night companion. Yet it is one worth pursuing because it comprises one third of the human life span. Use the Metabolic Matrix to adjust your nutrition, exercise regimen, and relaxation rituals, and identify the insights provided here on circadian rhythms to help you fall into a deep slumber. Well-timed, regular sleep habits are a form of metabolic enlightenment.

CHAPTER 12

Hormone Imbalances: A Few Cases of False Alarms

To know how to dissimulate is the knowledge of kings.
　　　　　　—Cardinal Richelieu, French statesman (1585–1642)

With insulin resistance, isolated measurements of certain hormones do not reflect their actual functional levels. Let us explain. Called serine protease inhibitors—often abbreviated to "serpins"—a super-class family of protein molecules comprised of as many as 350 amino acids exist in all life-forms.[1] Arising from common ancestral genes 600 million years ago, these protein molecules, of which there are more than 1,500 varieties, are found in humans, animals, roundworms, plants, fungi, viruses, and even bacteria. Without the inhibitory action of serpins, humans would be at risk for life-threatening blood clots, lethal tumors, endocrine disorders, and numerous other health issues.

Serpins, which have been compared to mousetraps, bind themselves to hormones and render them inactive. When insulin levels are higher than expected relative to the level of glucose, the effectiveness of the hormone regulation activity performed by serpin presence is reduced. This may lead to enhanced cortisol activity in children or increased testosterone levels and PCOS in women. The other serpin-related problem is that when doctors order standard lab tests of serpin-bound testosterone or thyroid hormone, instead of measuring the free amounts of the hormone that are biologically active and circulate in the blood, false results of hormone deficiency may appear because the amount of hormonally bound serpin is reduced and the serpin action is debilitated. These types of outcomes can lead physicians to make inappropriate medical decisions.

Distraught clients all too frequently appear at our clinic brandishing lab reports that purport to show that they have low thyroid levels or, in the case of men, abnormally low levels of testosterone. We reassure them that their hormone levels are likely to be normal but that their measurement is at fault. This phenomenon is one of the lesser understood facets (and, indeed, symptoms) of insulin resistance.[2]

LOW-T MYTHS

In June 1889, physician Charles-Édouard Brown-Séquard caused an uproar at the annual meeting of the *Société de Biologie* in Paris. He boasted that injections of "the elixir of life," or canine testicular extract, had endowed him with a second youth. Forty years later, at the University of Chicago, Professor Fred Koch and his coworkers collected tons of bull testicles from nearby slaughterhouses, extracting in the process—for the first time in human history—a few ounces of pure testosterone.

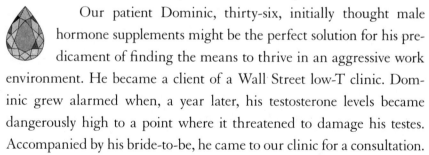
Our patient Dominic, thirty-six, initially thought male hormone supplements might be the perfect solution for his predicament of finding the means to thrive in an aggressive work environment. He became a client of a Wall Street low-T clinic. Dominic grew alarmed when, a year later, his testosterone levels became dangerously high to a point where it threatened to damage his testes. Accompanied by his bride-to-be, he came to our clinic for a consultation.

"Our office environment is very combative," he said. "People constantly yell at each other. The in-house competition never stops. In my world, nice guys finish last." Faced with these odds, Dominic sought help. "Last year, a couple of us at the office went to a low-T clinic favored by Wall Street traders. It offered the full hormonal suite of testosterone, HGH (human growth hormone); DHEA (dehydroepiandrosterone sulfate), plus vitamin D as prescription pills and injectables. I took testosterone shots for about a year. I was hitting all cylinders, able to concentrate for eight hours straight."

Dominic added, "Every week, the clinic sent a guy to check my blood. One of the tests came back showing my testosterone was through the roof. I began to read about how elevated levels could destroy my fertility. I am soon to be married and don't want to hurt myself or be unfair to my wife. We want children. So I have come to your clinic to seek immediate help."

With the plethora of ads touting treatments for low testosterone, it is important to know that there is a high rate of diagnostic errors in "low T" pronouncements, and men should not take testosterone supplements without close supervision. Too much testosterone can induce atrophy of the testes and lead to sterility.

Clinic Notes

At his initial consultation, Dominic carried 283 pounds on his five-foot-eleven frame, with a BMI of 39.0, high enough to be of medical concern. His testosterone levels (2,000 to 2,500 ng/ml) were two to three times the normal level. Once he stopped the testosterone supplements at our instruction, his levels fell to near 300, considered borderline low for a man of his age. In Dominic's case, as with many others that we see, this diagnosis of testosterone deficiency was incorrect. Dominic's high insulin blood levels had reduced the formation of SHBG (sex hormone-binding globulin), a type of serpin.[3]* This protein modifies the activities of steroid sex hormones, androgens, and estradiol by controlling their access to target cells. A central premise of endocrinology is that the biological effectiveness of hormones is determined by their "free" (non-protein-bound) concentrations.[4]

When the laboratory measures testosterone levels in the blood, most

---

* Testosterone largely circulates in the blood, bound to a protein known as sex hormone-binding globulin (SHBG), where it is rendered inactive and unable to bind to its intracellular receptors in testosterone-sensitive target cells.

of what is actually measured is, in fact, the testosterone bound to SHBG, where it is inert or inactive. Only 3 to 5 percent is believed to exist in a free (unbound) state, which has a biological effect. Many doctors do not realize that they would get a more accurate result if they had measured free or bioavailable testosterone levels, rather than total testosterone levels, in patients with insulin resistance. Indeed, when we tested Dominic's free testosterone level, we found it to be normal, even though his total testosterone levels were low.

Testosterone is a circadian hormone secreted during sleep. This means all men have the highest testosterone levels in the morning, hence their enhanced wakeful libido. If sleep is impaired by stress or sleep apnea before the blood for the test is drawn, the level is likely to be low even when testosterone secretions are not medically impaired. If a blood sample is taken in the afternoon, most men would be suspected of "low T."

WOMEN AND TESTOSTERONE

In the 1880s, when Madame Howard, the Lion-Faced Lady, was exhibited at a show in Britain's Lambeth Fair, her extravagant beard was ascribed to her English mother's carnal encounter with a lion in Sierra Leone. Hardly the truth. More recently, Mexican artist Frida Kahlo's self-portraits and lithographs have unforgettably immortalized her feathery mustache and her tragic miscarriage in 1932.[5]

The Thief of Parenthood

Dr. Irving F. Stein and his colleague Dr. Michael Leventhal first described a condition in which typically overweight women would develop excessive facial and bodily hair, experience menstrual irregularities, and develop ovarian cysts.[6]* Polycystic ovarian syndrome is

---

* There is a discrepancy between the NIH's 1990 diagnosis criteria, according to which a person must have all three of the symptoms of irregular ovulation, androgen excess,

estimated to affect 4 to 12 percent of all women of reproductive age.[7] In places such as India, PCOS affects as many as 26 percent of women in some communities.

Nainital Lake, India, where Nisha was born, is said to represent the eye of goddess Parvati, a place of cosmic power in Hindu mythology. As a child, Nisha was born small for her gestational age. "I faced a lot of family pressure and began seeing a psychiatrist for depression. Nor could I sleep. I do not believe I slept more than an hour at a time for two months."

Soon Nisha's menstrual cycle became erratic. Her mother, Urmila, treated her daughter with ancient Ayurvedic cures—teas of ginger, turmeric, and molasses. Regular outbreaks of acne followed. Nisha's once-thick, shoulder-length hair grew sparse.

Instead of following her plan of applying to schools in the United States for a PhD in human resources, at her mother's urging, Nisha created a profile on a matrimonial website. Meanwhile, on a Friday night in New Jersey, Suresh, a slim, shaggy-haired IT executive, responded to a friend's dare and wrote a few cheeky lines on the same website to "all the women out there." He immediately got a huffy response from Nisha. According to Suresh, "We began exchanging notes regularly." Six months later, they were married.

Five years later, Suresh said, "We've been through some tough times. At first, I could not understand how Nisha could eat a proper meal and be hungry again in an hour. Lately, as we have tried to start a family, Nisha gets so depressed at our failed attempts to have a child."

Clinic Notes

When we first saw Nisha, she was five feet two inches tall and weighed 188 pounds. Her family history indicated that her maternal grandmother had untreated type 2 diabetes and had died at age

---

and polycystic ovaries, and the Rotterdam definition (2003), which includes two of the three.

fifty-four. Nisha's aunt on her mother's side also had acute diabetes, lost her vision, and suffered from extremely high blood pressure.

Nisha's infrequent episodes of depression are a hallmark of insulin resistance, as was her tendency to be hungry soon after a large meal. Six weeks after she received her dietary guidelines, she had lost five pounds and looked more alert and happier. During the time when her body weight was erratic, Nisha had tried two cycles of fertility treatments that failed.

Two years later, on a regular clinic visit, Nisha reported that she was pregnant, but sadly, she miscarried at six weeks. Nisha had a classic case of polycystic ovarian syndrome, which results in increased levels of androgenic, or male, hormones. Half of those affected with this condition struggle with weight gain. In a woman, the pituitary gland accelerates the production of luteinizing hormone, which stimulates the ovaries to secrete increased amounts of testosterone. This often results in a failure of the ovaries to release an egg. Retention of eggs can lead to cyst formation. Furthermore, an excess of testosterone can produce other symptoms, all of which Nisha experienced: acne, loss of head hair, increased facial hair, missed menstrual periods, and infertility. Weight loss is beneficial to every aspect of PCOS.

Sometimes a woman can have normal levels of testosterone but still experience such symptoms. In such cases, the explanation is that the level of free and biologically available testosterone is high. This occurs because insulin resistance suppresses the formation of a serpin named SHBG, to which most of the testosterone in the circulation is bound and thereby inactivated.

After six years of yo-yo weight patterns, Nisha came to the MetaKura program, where our team monitored her closely. With a regular exercise regimen, a tailored diet, and medication, Nisha lost forty pounds, and the regularity of her menstrual periods improved. Nisha and Suresh now have a four-year-old daughter with a winning smile.

THE ENIGMA OF LOW THYROID FUNCTION

The reputation of the town of Iga Ueno, located near Osaka, has been assured by two men: Matsuo Bashō, one of Japan's most revered haiku poets, and the physician Hakaru Hashimoto. In 1912, at age thirty-one, Hashimoto published his discovery in *Archiv Für Klinishe Chirurgie,* a German journal, on an autoimmune thyroid condition in which a laggard, underperforming (hypo-) thyroid provokes puffiness, dry skin, disordered digestion, and muscle aches. Hypothyroidism affects one out of every thirty women worldwide.

"Crimes of passion may be traced in no small part to disturbances of the thyroid," wrote Louis Berman, in his 1921 bestseller, *The Glands Regulating Personality.* The mysterious thyroid gland, from which flows the largest number of the body's hormones (T3 and T4), offers a blueprint for sustained action. Thyroid hormones enter all cells of the body, wriggle into the driver's seat in receptors located in the cells' nuclei, and begin regulating the speed at which many functions of each cell operate. Thyroid hormones thyroxine (T4) and triiodothyronine (T3) are unbound, meaning that they traverse freely through cells, where they regulate the metabolism.

After the initial autoimmune assault, the thyroid is wooed back by the pituitary's thyroid-stimulating hormone (TSH) charm offensive, and its hormones hobble back to a normal range. However, as the collateral autoimmune damage accrues, thyroid supplements become necessary. As with the case of Dominic, most medical practitioners do not take into consideration that insulin resistance leads to a decline in the level of the transport serpin thyroid-binding globulin (TBG) in the blood. The result is a low level of thyroid hormones (but normal TSH because bioactive thyroid hormone levels are normal). This scenario often leads to an incorrect diagnosis of hypothyroidism (underactive thyroid).

When hypothyroidism is accurately diagnosed, and treated with thyroid hormone therapy, there is little to no weight loss. Once we confirm that an individual with hypothyroidism also has insulin resistance, we address both conditions in tandem with dietary changes and suggesting thyroid replacement medication when needed. Chronically neglected hypothyroidism can damage the heart, a condition called cardiomyopathy, or can lead to depression or even a form of psychosis known as myxedematous madness. In growing girls, hypothyroidism can retard growth (height) and sexual development.

CAN THIS DEFICIT BE FIXED?

In 1979, New York sizzled with labor unrest amid malodorous street corners piled high with uncollected garbage. "There's nothing better for building a six-year-old's self-confidence than standing in a picket line surrounded by angry adults," said Laura, forty-three, a biotech entrepreneur. With an engaging, friendly manner, she credits her father, a trade union leader, with her feisty spirit.

As a child, Laura crammed sailing, tennis, ballet, ice-skating, and competitive swimming into her after-school hours.

"I do remember being told in third or fourth grade that I did not have the right body profile for ballet," she said. "I guess I always had poor eating habits. Look, I'm up at six every morning and at my desk in the city by eight. Until six p.m., I give it my all."

A constant feature of Laura's adult life has been fluctuations in her dress size, resulting in a wardrobe that features clothes ranging from size 10 to size 14. Since joining the MetaKura program, after losing eleven pounds, she now finds the seat on her commuter train more comfortable. "The biggest change for me is in my mind. Thanks to the program, I have a mental filter that makes me pause to think about what I eat. I've swung open a kitchen cabinet door and then closed it twenty times looking at a piece of chocolate. Eventually, I decided that I would not bother. Earlier, I would have gone to a juice bar for a green shake; but now I read the sugar content more carefully.

"I do not aspire to be perfect. Perfect is such a terrible word," she added. "It's not my body size but my success that has been intimidating to some men. I know I can't be perfect every day. You have to be able to forgive yourself and not beat yourself up." Then she revealed that she has recently committed to a new boyfriend.

Clinic Notes

Laura was referred to the Clinic because of a thyroid enlargement that turned out to be Hashimoto's disease, a type of autoimmune thyroid disease. One of the first clues to Laura's weight gain was keratinocytes, basal cells found on the epidermis of the skin, especially around the eyelids, that react to elevated insulin levels by dispatching excessive amounts of a protein called keratin to these areas, akin to the protective bark of a tree.

One of the greatest misperceptions in medicine is that weight gain can be attributed to low thyroid levels. For women like Laura, high levels of insulin overpower the serpin, a major thyroid hormone transporter binding protein (thyroid binding globulin [TBG]) in the blood, thereby lowering the measurement of circulating thyroid hormone. This tricks the lab technician or medical practitioner into believing the hormone has all but disappeared. All the while, free and biologically available thyroid hormone may be present in normal quantities. However, in Laura's case, her unbound (free T4) level was low.

Indeed, even as her thyroid function normalized with medication, Laura continued to experience metabolism-related complications. She was found to have dyslipidemia (elevated triglyceride levels and low HDL cholesterol), which is typical of someone with insulin dysfunction. In her case, as with many others, the excess insulin was increasing the size of her fat cells.

Recent research has shown that serpins may also be a culprit in the development of the fastest growing disease in the elderly. Studies of Alzheimer's patients have found an increased presence of specific serpins* in their cerebrospinal fluid. Furthermore, in a mouse model of the disease, the expression of serpins greatly increased the amyloid-precursor proteins into classic Alzheimer's-like plaques in the brain.

---

* Neuroserpin alpha (1) anti-chymotrypsin and alpha (1) anti-trypsin

In conclusion, although we have presented a number of instances illustrating how serpins can sow confusion and even risk, it is important to understand that they also provide therapeutic benefits, cancer therapies, improved gluten tolerance, and treatment for hemophilia. Our gut microbiome hosts 32 percent of the known serpin population. For all these reasons, continued research into these serpin tricksters is critical. Deciphering their subtle capabilities is now seen as a promising route to new therapies for healing.

PART III

The Protocol

CHAPTER 13

Match Your Food Plan to Your Metabolism

Congratulations on taking your first bold step! The philosophy of the MetaKura program is to give you the knowledge that you will need to be firmly in charge of your physical and mental well-being. Focus on the vast range of foods that you *can* enjoy. Know that as you follow the steps recommended in this book, you will have so much more energy that you will not want to go back to your old ways.

Tips for designing your plan to balance your metabolism:

- Keep in mind that because your metabolism is dynamic, you can use the Metabolic Matrix and the MetaKura food guidelines to improve your profile over time. For example, like so many of our patients on the MetaKura program, you may start out with a Ruby personality (insulin resistance with medical complications) and in six months' time, when your blood sugar, hypertension, and cholesterol are within the normal range, progress to an Emerald personality (insulin resistance with symptoms and no overt medical complications). Or you may improve from an Emerald personality with symptoms like chronic fatigue, hair loss, or poor sleep patterns to a Sapphire personality (asymptomatic insulin resistance). You are in charge of driving this change.

- Focus on substitution instead of restriction. If you crave a certain food, use our recommended food list to come up with creative alternatives. Replace potato chips with parmesan zucchini chips or wheat-based spaghetti with lentil-made pasta.

- Because this is a lifelong program, be kind to yourself if you have slipups. Get back on track the next day. If you are tempted to eat dessert, have one or two spoonfuls, no more.
- The MetaKura food guidelines have been adapted to many global cuisines. People have proudly told us that they were able to adhere to their dietary guidelines on two-week-long family road trips, at religious observances across faiths, through the temptations of the holiday season, and even on extended vacations on cruise ships.
- Carry a recommended snack with you at all times. This is an important element in maintaining your insulin stability on the program. You should always have the right foods nearby in case you get hungry.

While the program is very flexible and each profile has latitude in the foods they can eat, there are some foods that should be avoided.

Not Recommended for Any MetaKura Personality Type

- Ice cream—unless zero sugar.
- Pizza and pasta—best avoided unless the pizza base is 100 percent cauliflower. Pasta is permitted if the only ingredient is lentil flour.
- Prepared food: check ingredients for added sugar, sugar alcohol, rice flour, tapioca, agave, and other ingredients that are not part of your food list.
- Processed food (sold in packages and cans): best avoided unless they contain simple, natural ingredients.

Making these changes in your diet alone will help you in improving your health.

THE JADE PERSONALITY PROFILE
RECOMMENDED FOOD LIST AND
METABOLISM GUIDELINES

Eat Freely	Eat Occasionally (2–3 times a month if not specified)	Eat Rarely (once every month)
Vegetables: most accepted	Squash, yam, taro, pumpkin	Potatoes, beets
Fruits: Granny Smith apples, all berries, pears, plums, nectarines	Figs, corn, apples: ½ cup per week	Dried fruit, pineapple, watermelon, grapes, bananas, mangoes, oranges, all coconut-based products
Tofu products		Seitan (gluten product)
All beans and legumes	Sweetened chocolate (1 small bar per week)	Chocolate that is less than 75 percent cacao
Herbs and spices, all types	Premade spice mixes with less than 5 mg of sugar	Spices with added sugar
Nuts and seeds, all types Almond and other nut-based milk (unsweetened) Nut-based flour	Nuts with flavoring that may contain sugar	Nut butter with added sugar
Olive oil	Ghee and butter	Canola, avocado, macadamia oil
Spelt, buckwheat, steel-cut oats, millet, quinoa*	Whole grains: ½ cup per week	Cornmeal, rye, tapioca, rice, wheat, maize, barley, amaranth, teff
Eggs, cheese, plain Greek yogurt, ricotta cheese	Milk, butter	Milk shakes, flavored yogurt, ice cream
Fish, shellfish, mollusks	Prepared seafood salads (may have added sugar)	Seafood in sauces with added sugar
Poultry of all types	Rotisserie chicken (may have added sugar)	Wheat batter–fried chicken
Lean meats	Meats: beef, lamb, pork, veal, venison, goat	Meats prepared with sugar or brine

(continue)

Eat Freely	Eat Occasionally (2–3 times a month if not specified)	Eat Rarely (once every month)
Monk fruit powder, stevia	Honey: 1 tsp twice a week	Sugar, molasses, agave, sugar alcohols
Condiments or seasoning with no sugar	Condiments or seasoning (less than 5 g of sugar)	Ketchup, barbecue sauce, rice vinegar
Tea, coffee, unsweetened cocoa, sparkling water, vegetable juice (with no added sugar)	Red wine, vodka: 2–3 glasses per week (sugar-free mixers)	Fruit juices (including berry juice), smoothies with high glycemic fruits, cocktails

*Quinoa offers essential amino acids for vegans and vegetarians, though it should be eaten in small quantities.

Diet

Jades should opt for small, frequent meals. All sugars, sucrose (table sugars and sweetened food), glucose (bread and pasta), fructose (fruits, some vegetables, honey), and lactose (milk products), place the heaviest load on the metabolism, especially in terms of mental clarity.

Exercise

Jades should engage in cardiovascular exercise, such as walking, yoga, taking fitness classes, or participate in fitness routines at a gym at least three times per week. Exercising more frequently is more desirable, although overall consistency in one's routine is the most advisable. Exercise also promotes energy, emotional well-being, and mental health. Find a level of intensity that is comfortable for you and commit to making it part of your daily or weekly routine.

Sleep

The reason for getting six to eight hours of sleep per day is that lack of sleep is one of the most common reasons for metabolic imbalances.

Vital hormones such as cortisol, testosterone, and growth hormone are released at night during periods of deep sleep.

THE SAPPHIRE PERSONALITY PROFILE RECOMMENDED FOOD LIST AND METABOLISM GUIDELINES

Eat Freely	Eat Occasionally (1–2 times a month)	Eat Rarely (once a month)
Vegetables: most accepted	Pumpkin, butternut squash	Potatoes, beets, squash, yam, taro
Fruits: Granny Smith apples, all berries, crunchy pears, firm plums	Crunchy apricots and nectarines	Dried fruit, pineapple, watermelon, grapes, bananas, oranges, figs, pears, apples, mangoes. Avoid fruit juice.
Soy and unprocessed protein meat substitutes	Seitan	Sweetened soy products
All beans and legumes	Lentil pasta (100 percent lentils): once per week	Chocolate that is less than 75 percent cacao
Herbs and spices, all types	Prepared spice mixes	Spices with added sugar
Nuts and seeds, all types Almond flour and other nut-based flour	Nut bars or butter with 5+ g of added sugar	Nut-based snack bars or butter with 6+ g of added sugar
Olive, canola, avocado, macadamia oil	Ghee and butter	Margarine, coconut oil
Spelt, buckwheat, steel-cut oats, bulgur 2–3 servings per week	Millet or quinoa (the latter is beneficial for vegans/vegetarians)	Cornmeal, rye, tapioca, rice, wheat, maize, barley, sorghum, teff, amaranth
Eggs, cheese (all types), plain Greek yogurt, ricotta, unsweetened almond milk	Butter, milk, plain yogurt (½ cup twice per week)	Milk shakes, flavored yogurt
Fish, shellfish, mollusks	Prepared seafood salads (may have added sugar)	Seafood in sauces with added sugar

(continue)

Eat Freely	Eat Occasionally (1–2 times a month)	Eat Rarely (once a month)
Poultry, all types	Rotisserie chicken (may have added sugar)	Batter-fried chicken, any poultry with barbecue or other sauces that may contain sugar
Lean meats	Meats: beef, lamb, pork, veal, venison, goat	Meats prepared with sugar, including cold cuts
All 100 percent vegetable pasta like zucchini spaghetti	Pastas made with almond flour	Pizza, pasta, baked goods
Monk fruit powder, stevia		Sugar, molasses, honey, agave, sugar alcohols
Condiments, seasoning (sugar-free)	Unsweetened chili or other sauces	Ketchup, barbecue sauce
Tea, coffee, unsweetened cocoa, sparkling water, vegetable juice (with no added sugar)	Red wine, vodka (with sugar-free mixers): 2–3 glasses per week	Fruit juices (including berry juice), smoothies with high glycemic fruits, cocktails

Diet

Sapphires should eat small meals every two to three hours. It is important to plan your weekly meals and snacks. Sapphires should be mindful about hidden ingredients in their food, especially when they dine at restaurants, purchase prepared food, or are on the road. Check labels and ask your server so you can avoid sugar or simple carbohydrate ingredients. Fiber-rich nuts and prebiotic cabbage, leeks, and other foods are your dietary friends. Protein will give you a sense of satiety. Leafy and raw vegetables will help your digestion. For you, complex carbohydrates (beans, steel-cut oats) are always preferable.

Sapphires should switch to a high-fiber diet and strictly limit high glycemic foods, including rice, sugar, breads, pasta, milk, flavored yogurts, plantain, corn syrup, and sugar alcohols. They should be generally mindful of avoiding foods with all types of sugar. Sucrose (table sugars and sweetened foods), glucose (bread and pasta), fructose (fruits, some vegetables, honey), and lactose (milk products) should be restricted. Sapphires should avoid large meals comprised of dense calorie foods, as well as most grains. Focus on distinguishing between simple and complex carbohydrates such as lentils, beans, and complex grains like buckwheat or millet, where the latter have longer chains of sugar molecules and therefore glucose does not enter the bloodstream so quickly. Be alert to so-called healthy foods such as brown rice, beets, and coconut water, which place an especially heavy load on a Sapphire metabolism and have been implicated in degrading brain network stability over time.

Although ketogenic diets (low carb and high fat) have been found to be beneficial for reducing blood glucose levels and enabling weight loss, many people find them challenging to sustain long term.

Exercise

In addition to making mindful selections for your diet, exercise is the best gift that you can give your body. A regular cardio exercise routine is also a must, at a minimum of three and preferably five days a week. Your choice of physical activity can be gentle like walking or yoga, but it should be of sufficient duration (forty-five to sixty minutes) and regularity to make a difference. This type of exercise makes a dramatic change in enabling glucose to act more effectively in your muscles, to give you more vitality. For those being treated for anxiety or depression, exercise has been shown to be extremely beneficial.

Sleep

A minimum of seven hours of sleep is essential for your health and the normal functioning of your nocturnal hormones. Keep in mind that sleep deprivation increases craving for comfort foods and reduces your glucose sensitivity, meaning that it will promote accumulation of fat stores in your body. Lack of sleep is one of the most common reasons for metabolism-related imbalances because vital hormones such as cortisol, testosterone, and growth hormone are released at night during periods of deep sleep.

THE EMERALD PERSONALITY PROFILE RECOMMENDED FOOD LIST AND METABOLISM GUIDELINES

Eat Freely	Eat Occasionally (once a month)	Eat Rarely (once in 3 months)
Vegetables: most accepted other than the ones on the right columns	Spaghetti squash, parsnips, peas	Potatoes, beets, squash, yam, taro, pumpkin, corn
Fruits: Granny Smith apples, all berries	Plums and crunchy pears (1–2 fruits per week)	Dried fruit, pineapple, watermelon, grapes
All beans and legumes	Lentil pasta (made with 100 percent lentils) once per week	Chocolate that is less than 75 percent cacao
Herbs and spices, all types		Spices with added sugar
Nuts and seeds, all types	Nut bars or nut butter with 3 g or less of added sugar	Nut bars or butter with 6+ g of added sugar
Almond flour and other nut flours		
Almond milk and other nut-based milks (unsweetened)		
Olive oil	Ghee and butter	Canola, avocado, macadamia
	Limit spelt, buckwheat, steel-cut oats to 1–2 servings per week of one of these. Soba noodles (if buckwheat is the only ingredient)	Cornmeal, rye, tapioca, rice, wheat, maize, barley
Eggs, cheese, plain Greek yogurt, ricotta cheese	Butter	Milk shakes, flavored yogurt

Fish, shellfish, mollusks	Prepared seafood salads (may have added sugar)	Seafood in sauces with added sugar
Poultry, all types	Rotisserie chicken (may have added sugar)	Deli preparations
Lean meats	Meats: beef, lamb, pork, veal, venison, goat	Meats prepared with sugar, including cold cuts
Soy, edamame, and unprocessed protein meat substitutes	Processed meat substitutes	Seitan (gluten product)
Stevia, monk fruit sweetener		Sugar, molasses, honey, agave, sugar alcohols
Condiments	Prepared seasoning (less than 5 g of sugar)	Ketchup, barbecue sauce, rice vinegar
Tea, coffee, unsweetened cocoa, sparkling water, vegetable juice (with no added sugar)	Red wine, plain vodka (2–3 glasses per week with sugar-free mixers)	Fruit juices (including berry juice), smoothies with high glycemic fruits, cocktails

Diet

Emeralds can do wonders for their sense of well-being by being vigilant about their food choices. For this reason, Emeralds should become nutritional sleuths who check the ingredients of everything, whether in restaurants, cafés, grocery stores, or online takeout so they can avoid most grain and sugar altogether. Our recipes are quick and simple because the more that you are able to cook for yourself, the more you will be in charge of the metabolism-friendly nutrition going into your body. Remember, we do not believe in counting calories or restricting portions, so you should never, ever be hungry on this program. Also certain kinds of food—most granola, baked goods, and wraps (unless made with MetaKura-permitted grains)—are hunger-creating foods. Including daily combinations of high-fiber foods, micronutrients found in fresh vegetables, and healthy proteins will make your metabolism (and you) sing.

Emeralds should be more watchful of the simple sugars in their diet than Sapphires. You can enjoy unlimited quantities of most vegetables, berries, nuts, and seeds, as well as a wide variety of proteins. You should be highly observant and ask your server when you dine in restaurants about added sugars, and review labels carefully on packaged items that you purchase in a supermarket. Processed snacks, rice flour, coconut-based products, and sugar alcohols are best avoided. Focus on simplicity, freshness, and plenty of the right types of foods that are identified in your meal plan. We are more interested in the nutritional properties of food and your body's responses to your choice of sustenance. It is advisable for Emeralds to carry snacks with them to keep their insulin levels stable. The degree to which you will need to closely monitor your meal plans will depend on the acuteness of your condition, but the changes must be permanent.

Exercise

Targeted physical activities help glucose act more effectively in your muscles. Exercise also helps support emotional well-being and mental health. Find a level of intensity that is comfortable for you and commit to making it part of your daily routine. Walk at least three miles and build up to ten thousand steps every day or engage in other forms of more rigorous exercise if you are able. (Our ancestors apparently walked an average of nine hours a day!) We recommend you engage in cardio exercise at least five days a week, as vigorously as you can, and more often if you are also suffering from fatigue or depression. This may seem illogical, but we have seen it be highly effective to relieve those conditions.

Sleep

Get six to eight hours per night. Check that you do not snore or that you do not stop breathing while asleep (obstructive sleep apnea), as this affects glucose sensitivity, which in turn increases the risk of unwanted weight gain. A number of our patients have cured their sleep apnea after correcting their metabolic health. Interrupted or insufficient sleep is one of the most common reasons for chronic metabolism imbalances. Vital hormones such as cortisol, testosterone, and growth hormone are released at night during deep sleep. Disturbed sleep patterns are also a primary cause of hypertension.

THE RUBY PERSONALITY PROFILE RECOMMENDED FOOD LIST AND METABOLISM GUIDELINES

Eat Freely	Eat Occasionally (once a month)	Eat Rarely (once in 3 months)
Vegetables: most accepted	Spaghetti squash	Beets, squash, yam, taro, pumpkin, parsnips, corn
Granny Smith apples, all berries		All other fruit including dried fruit and fruit juices
All beans and legumes	Chickpeas and other legumes once or twice per week	Chocolate that is less than 75 percent cacao
Pasta made with 100 percent lentil flour		
Herbs and spices	Limit salt with food if recommended by your doctor.	Spices with added sugar
	Prepared spices with less than 3 g sugar	
Nuts and seeds, all types	Nut bars or nut butter with 4 g or less of added sugar (1–2 per servings per week)	Nut bars or butter with 6+ g of added sugar, honey-roasted or those with corn syrup or cornstarch in the ingredients
Almond flour and other pure nut-based flour		
Nut butters with no added sugar		
Unsweetened almond milk		
Olive, avocado, macadamia oil	Ghee and butter. Limit fried food.	Margarine, coconut oil

(continue)

Eat Freely	Eat Occasionally (once a month)	Eat Rarely (once in 3 months)
Nut-based flour and seed-flour	Limit spelt, buckwheat, steel-cut oats to ½ cup of one of these, every ten days.	Cornmeal, rye, tapioca, rice, wheat, maize, barley, teff, amaranth
Eggs, plain Greek yogurt, fresh or pressed uncooked cheese, ricotta	Butter, Parmesan, Fontina, Gouda cheese	Milk or yogurt, blue cheese, bloomy cheese
Fish, shellfish, mollusks	Prepared seafood salads (may have added sugar)	Seafood in sauces with added sugar
Poultry, all types	Rotisserie chicken (may have added sugar)	Deli chicken made with brine, maple
Lean meats	Meats: beef, lamb, pork, veal, venison, goat	Meats prepared with sugar, including cold cuts
Soy and unprocessed protein meat substitutes	Seitan (gluten product)	No meat substitutes with processed ingredients
Monk fruit powder, stevia, monk fruit sweetener		Sugar, molasses, honey, agave, sugar alcohols
Condiments and seasoning with no added sugar	Premade salad dressing and sauces (less than 3 g of sugar)	Ketchup, barbecue sauce
Tea, coffee, unsweetened cocoa, sparkling water, vegetable juice (with no added sugar)	Red wine, vodka: 1–2 glasses per week with sugar-free mixers. Limit diet sodas.	Fruit juices (including berry juice), smoothies with high glycemic fruits, cocktails

Diet

Ruby personalities have a medical diagnosis. We therefore recommend discussing any dietary or lifestyle changes with your physician. Avoid blood sugar highs and lows by eating small amounts regularly and carrying snacks with you. Our most important message for you is that by following these guidelines, we believe that you can be a champion for your health and do wonders to reverse your medical complications.

As a first step, Rubies should be kinder to their bodies' need to produce excessive insulin by *strictly* eliminating all insulin-spiking foods such as rice, sugar, and flour. Our recipes are simple, quick, and incredibly delicious. Remember that we do not believe in counting calories or restricting portions. If you enjoy ethnic cuisines, you can still enjoy them by substituting ingredients. Over time, this protocol will lower your levels of blood lipids (triglycerides) and blood glucose. Ruby, get inspiration from so many of our patients who rejoice in their new health. Your goals are achievable and the benefits to you are immeasurable. Take charge now.

Exercise

Contrary to common beliefs, overweight people have a high rather than a low resting energy expenditure, but the metabolism slows with weight loss as the body attempts to regain its former weight (homeostasis). The best way to counter this rebound effect is with regular exercise—the more vigorous, the better.

Walk at least three miles *every* day or engage in other forms of more rigorous exercise if your health allows. If you are also suffering from fatigue or depression, we have seen daily exercise to be highly effective. Exercise makes insulin act more efficiently in your muscles, so you feel less tired.

Sleep

Get seven to eight hours a day. Be sure that you don't snore or have obstructive sleep apnea. A lack of sleep or poor-quality sleep is a primary cause of excess weight gain, as it reduces glucose sensitivity and promotes fat stores in the body. Vital hormones such as cortisol, testosterone, and growth hormone are released at night during periods of deep sleep. Over time, as the body's ability to regulate these stress hormones declines, your risk for high blood pressure increases.

Now you are ready to start. We believe that you will do wonders!

CHAPTER 14

Getting Started: Recommendations for Your Kitchen and Pantry

With the MetaKura way of life, we celebrate food that has been freshly grown from the earth as an expression of our primal connection with the natural world. We take pleasure in nourishing our minds and our bodies with a cornucopia of vegetables, fruits, proteins, and fibers, rich in flavors and micronutrients. Knowing the properties of specific foods, we think of them as healing tonics to boost energy, improve cognition, or to soothe digestion. We approach the dazzling flavors of fresh, pure, and simple nutrition every day, confident in the knowledge of which foods are friendliest to each one of our unique metabolisms. Recently, a client brought to our attention that the MetaKura program is environmentally friendly, because by relying primarily on fresh foods, few food purchases necessitate plastic containers or cans.

Before you can start putting nourishing food into your body, you need to get the unhealthy food out of your home and out of your life. We will walk you through the categories of foods that should no longer be found in your kitchen and give you information on how to fill your grocery bags and shelves—and your plate—with healthy alternatives. (See Chapter 13 for specifics on foods for your metabolism personality.)

A DETOX FOR YOUR PANTRY

Clear out foods with ingredients that contain even traces of grains other than spelt, millet, and buckwheat. Remove any products with more than four grams of sugar per serving, including sugar alcohols like sorbitol, mannitol, and erythritol. This includes all types of sauces, condiments, and prepared salad dressing. Coconut-based products contain harmful fats, so bid them farewell.

Foods to Remove

Proteins: Deli meats (prepared or brined in sugar or sauces), maple turkey, bacon, or ham

Vegetables: Beets, potatoes, squash (except spaghetti squash), sweet potatoes, cassava

Dairy: Milk, ice cream, standard yogurt

Grains: Amaranth, cornmeal, farro, millet, tapioca, wheat flour

Fruits: Red apples, bananas, cherry, coconut, date, figs, fruit juices, grapes, kiwi, mango, melon, nectarines (ripe), oranges, papaya, peaches (ripe), pineapple

Snacks and drinks: Cake, cookies, pastries, pretzels, chips (unless made with ingredients like almond flour or monk fruit powder), sodas, all fruit juices, sweet tea, sugar

Once you have cleared your shelves, refrigerator, and kitchen of the foods that will not support your new way of eating, it's time to fill up with healthy alternatives!

A RESTOCK FOR YOUR PANTRY

Health for Your Shelf

Oils: Olive, ghee (avoid coconut oil)

Grains (recommended in moderation): Buckwheat, spelt, millet, steel-cut oats

Beans and Legumes: All types are encouraged. Beans, lentils, chickpeas, edamame, tofu, and hummus. (This includes pastas but only if made with 100 percent lentils.)

Nuts and Seeds: We champion all varieties of seeds and nuts, provided they have no added sugars, including almonds, cashews, chestnuts, chai seeds, flax seeds, hazelnuts, pecans, pine nuts, pistachios, pumpkin seeds, sunflower seeds, and walnuts. Also choose nut flours like almond, macadamia, and walnut flour. Seed crackers (with permissible ingredients) are permitted.

Beverages: Unsweetened teas, especially mint (soothing), cocoa powder (antioxidants), turmeric (anti-inflammatory), coffee

Condiments and vinegars: All types of sugar-free condiments are acceptable, including ketchup, hot sauce, all mustards, and all vinegar except rice vinegar.

Canned items: Tomatoes, artichokes, olives, and others on your metabolism personality food list

Sweeteners: Monk fruit powder, stevia, sugar substitutes, excluding agave

Recommended Fresh Produce and Proteins

Vegetables

- arugula, artichokes, asparagus, avocado
- bok choy, broccoli, Brussels sprouts
- cabbage, carrots, cauliflower, celery, chives, collard greens, cucumber
- dill
- eggplant, endive
- frisee (endive)
- garlic, green beans, ginger
- haricots verts
- kale, kohlrabi
- leeks, lettuce

- mixed greens, mushrooms, mustard greens
- okra, onions
- parsley, peppers
- radicchio, radish, romaine lettuce
- snap peas, spaghetti squash, spinach, sprouts, shallots, Swiss chard
- tomatoes, turnips
- watercress
- zucchini

Vegetables in moderation: peas and corn

Herbs and spices (fresh or dried)

- anise
- basil
- caraway, coriander (also known as cilantro), chamomile
- dill
- fennel
- lavender, lemon grass
- marjoram
- oregano
- parsley
- rosemary
- sage
- thyme

Fruits

- apricot
- berries: blackberries, blueberries, raspberries, strawberries
- Granny Smith apples
- green pears (Jade, Sapphire personalities)
- lemon and lime
- plum (unripe only)

Proteins

Dairy: Cheese (all types), Greek yogurt (plain, fat content of choice)

Dairy substitutes: Almond milk (unsweetened), soy milk (unsweetened)

Eggs: All types

Fish: Salmon, sole, flounder, sea bass, tuna, and others; shellfish (shrimp, crabs, lobster, crayfish, and others); mollusks (clam, oyster, squid, and others)

Poultry: Chicken, turkey, duck

Meat: Beef, pork, lamb (if you are an omnivore)

Meat substitutes: Avoid all products with ultra-processed ingredients and added beets

KITCHEN ESSENTIALS

A well-equipped kitchen makes preparing meals on the MetaKura plan easy. Stocking your kitchen should be fun, as you only need a few basics to start making delicious meals at home. The following recommendations assume that you are starting from scratch. You may already have many of the items, so simply add what you need. Look for well-made products with good reviews, and you can't go wrong.

Cookware

Stainless steel is best. You are often able to find a complete set.

- 8-quart stockpot with cover
- 3-quart saucepan with cover
- 3-quart sauté pan with cover
- 1½-quart saucepan with cover
- 10-inch skillet

- 1 nonstick skillet, 8-inch or 10-inch
- cast iron grill or skillet

Kitchen Utensils

Stainless-steel utensils are great but will scratch nonstick cookware, so investing in some silicone utensils is a good idea.

- colander
- cutting board
- spoon
- slotted spoon
- tongs
- spatula
- silicone spatula
- whisk
- wooden spoons

Appliances

Bearing in mind that all the recipes can be prepared the old-fashioned way with a knife and a cutting board, some electric appliances will definitely save a lot of prep time.

Food processor: Will quickly chop, grind, grate, and slice. Used mostly for dry ingredients. There are many brands available at a range of price points. It's a great appliance to have and definitely makes prep work a breeze. If you are only going to buy one appliance, buy this one.

Blender: Is great for making salad dressings, marinades—anything liquid. If your budget allows for a top-of-the-line, high-speed blender, that's great. You will also get great results with a

NutriBullet, which is a small, inexpensive personal blender, with several cups; one version comes with a millet blade that can be used to grind nuts, coffee, and spices.

Immersion blender: Is an inexpensive tool that is great for puréeing soups and blending salad dressings and marinades.

Instant Pot: Several recipes call for a slow cooker, which allows you to place all the ingredients in it, set it, and go, and when you return home, your meal is ready and warm, waiting for you. The Instant Pot is recommended because in addition to the slow cooker function, it is a pressure cooker, steamer, sauté pan, and yogurt maker. You can also opt for a traditional slow cooker.

Dash egg cooker: A very inexpensive device that makes hard- and soft-boiled eggs, poached eggs, and omelets, without you being in the room. You put the eggs in, set it and go, and return to perfect eggs every time. It is highly recommended.

Knives

You should buy the best knives you can afford. Whatever you buy, wash them by hand, dry them, and store them in a block if possible. Never put them in the dishwasher. Keep them sharp with a honing steel before regular use. You can buy a number of different knives, but the ones you will rely on are:

- 6- or 8-inch chef's knife
- paring knife
- serrated knife

Gadgets

These are little tools that definitely make prep and cooking easier. Investing in something of a higher quality means you probably won't have to replace it.

- garlic press
- handheld citrus squeezer
- measuring spoons
- measuring cups (dry)
- measuring cups (liquid)
- meat thermometer
- salad spinner
- vegetable peeler

CHAPTER 15

Recipes for the MetaKura Program

BREAKFAST

Ricotta Pancake with Blueberry Compote
Avocado Toast
Blueberry and Avocado Smoothie Bowl
Cacio e Pepe Scrambled Eggs
Faux Açai Bowl
Yogurt Flax Pancakes with Raspberry Compote

SOUPS

Classic Vegetable Minestrone Soup
Chilled Avocado Soup
French Lentil Soup
Gazpacho
Spicy Slow-Cooked Black Bean Soup
Zucchini Curry Bisque

SALADS

Deviled Eggs over Baby Spinach with Green Goddess Dressing
Lemony Zucchini Salad
Curry Chicken Salad in Lettuce Cups
Pasta Salad with Avocado and Chicken
Smoked Salmon Rollups over Mixed Baby Greens

ENTRÉES

Whole Roasted Cauliflower with Herb Sauce
Grilled Shrimp Piccata
Pan-Roasted Salmon with Dill
Chicken Cutlets with Shallots and Capers
Spice-Rubbed Spatchcocked Chicken
Garam Masala Lamb Chops
Puerto Rican Pernil Pork Chops
Spiced Lamb Ragu
Citrus Skirt Steak with Chimichurri

ACCOMPANIMENTS/SIDES

Aglio e Olio
Cauliflower Purée
Haricots Verts with Mushroom and Shallots
Pinto Beans Sofrito
Homemade Sofrito
Herb-Roasted Spaghetti Squash

SAUCES

Puttanesca Sauce
Quick Marinara Sauce

DESSERTS

Chocolate Ricotta Mousse
Raspberry Ricotta Mousse
Poached Pears with Vanilla Sauce

BREAKFAST

Ricotta Pancake with Blueberry Compote

Serves 1
Active time: 5 minutes
Total time: 15 minutes

Jade and Sapphire (original recipe)
Emerald and Ruby (use fresh blueberries instead of compote)

A quick, delicious, healthy pancake with a warm compote. It's a recipe for one person that can easily be doubled or tripled for your whole family. You can prepare the compote ahead of time and keep it warm until ready to serve.

Pancake:

¼ cup part-skim ricotta

2 tablespoons ground flaxseed

1 teaspoon granulated monk fruit sweetener

½ teaspoon baking powder

1 large egg

½ teaspoon vanilla extract

Pinch of kosher salt

1 teaspoon butter

Whisk together the ricotta, ground flaxseed, monk fruit sweetener, baking powder, egg, vanilla extract, and salt in a small bowl. Heat an 8-inch nonstick skillet over medium heat. Melt the butter in the skillet, swirling to coat the pan, and then add the ricotta mixture, smoothing it with the back of a spoon into a round pancake. Lower the heat and allow to cook until golden brown, 4 to 5 minutes. Flip the pancake and cook an additional 2 to 4 minutes until golden and cooked through. Serve with compote on top.

Compote:

½ cup fresh or frozen blueberries

1 tablespoon fresh lemon juice

1 teaspoon granulated monk fruit sweetener

½ teaspoon ground cinnamon

½ teaspoon vanilla extract

Combine the berries, lemon juice, monk fruit sweetener, cinnamon, and vanilla in a small saucepan. Mash the berries using a potato masher. Heat the mixture over medium-low heat until simmering. Allow to simmer for 3 to 5 minutes or until slightly thickened and jam-like. Set aside and keep warm.

Avocado Toast

Serves 1
Active time: 10 minutes
Total time: 10 minutes

Jade (unrestricted)
Sapphire (up to three times per week)
Emerald (one toast, twice a week)
Ruby (one serving a week, though Ezekiel bread is best avoided)

With this simple recipe, the trickiest part is freeing the avocado flesh from its skin. To do that, place the avocado lengthwise on a cutting board and, while holding the top securely with one hand, slice slowly down the center lengthwise around the stone. Holding the avocado in the palm of one hand, use your other hand to twist and rotate the two halves apart. You can remove the stone by gently tapping it with the blade of a knife and working it out. To remove the fruit from the skin, use a spoon to scoop it out.

1 avocado, pitted and peeled

1 teaspoon olive oil

1 tablespoon freshly squeezed lemon juice

Red pepper flakes, to taste

Kosher salt, to taste

Paprika, to garnish

1 slice Ezekiel bread, or bread with 100 percent spelt flour or buckwheat

Poached egg (optional)

Using a fork, mash the avocado until smooth. Stir in the olive oil and lemon juice. Season with the kosher salt and red pepper flakes.

Toast the Ezekiel bread. Pile the mashed avocado mixture on top. Sprinkle with paprika and serve.

If serving with poached egg, make a small well in the mashed avocado and place the egg in the center.

For the Poached Egg:

Bring a small saucepan of water to a light boil. Crack the egg into a small strainer and allow the extra liquid white to drain off.

Using a slotted spoon, make a circular motion in the water to make a whirlpool effect. Add the egg carefully and allow the egg to spin. Cook for 3 to 4 minutes, gently spinning the water if it stops.

Remove the egg to a cool bath of water and hold in the water until ready to serve. If you would like to reheat the egg, just drop back into boiling water for a couple of seconds.

Blueberry and Avocado Smoothie Bowl

Serves 2
Active time: 10 minutes
Total time: 10 minutes

Jade, Sapphire, Emerald, and Ruby

(Note: Smoothies should not be regular substitutes for meals.)

A high-fiber smoothie bowl can be an occasional treat. You can create any combo of flavors and add toppings. It's far more satisfying than a regular smoothie because you can't just down it in ten seconds—you have to use a spoon! This recipe gives you the basics, but you can be creative and change up the fruits, greens, and nuts.

1 cup packed fresh spinach

1 cup fresh or frozen blueberries

½ avocado, pitted and peeled

⅓ to ½ cup unsweetened almond milk

1 tablespoon almond butter

2 tablespoons fresh lemon juice

1 (1-inch) piece fresh ginger, peeled and sliced

2 scoops protein powder (recommend Vega Protein & Greens, 30 grams, 120 calories)

Cold water, as necessary (can be adjusted based on desired consistency)

Garnish:

Sliced almonds

Fresh berries

Add the spinach, blueberries, avocado, almond milk, almond butter, lemon juice, ginger, and protein powder to the carafe of a high-speed blender. Blend until very smooth. Pour into two bowls and garnish with sliced almonds and berries as desired.

Cacio e Pepe Scrambled Eggs

Serves 1
Active time: 10 minutes
Total time: 10 minutes

Jade, Sapphire, Emerald, and Ruby

The translation of *cacio e pepe* is cheese and pepper. Made with a thick spaghetti called *tonnarelli*, Pecorino Romano, and black pepper, this cheesy pasta dish has been a staple of Roman cuisine for decades. This take on the classic pasta dish changes your everyday scrambled eggs into a little taste of Italy. *Buon appetito.*

2 large eggs

1 teaspoon water

2 tablespoons grated Pecorino Romano cheese

1 teaspoon grated black pepper

Kosher salt, to taste

2 teaspoons extra-virgin olive oil

Whisk the eggs and water together in a bowl until well combined. Stir in the cheese and black pepper. Season with salt, to taste. Heat the olive oil over low heat in a nonstick skillet. Add the egg mixture and cook, stirring constantly with a rubber spatula, until small curds begin to form and the eggs are cooked through, 4 to 5 minutes, and serve.

This can be served with a slice of toasted Ezekiel bread or some crisped pancetta for Jade and Sapphire.

Faux-Açai Bowl

Serves 1
Active time: 15 minutes
Total time: 15 minutes

Jade, Sapphire, Emerald, and Ruby

The ever-popular açai bowl is off limits on the MetaKura program due to the high sugar content of the ingredients used to prepare it. This delicious, healthy rendition takes advantage of all the health benefits of açai while forgoing the excess sugar. Due to increasing recognition and demand, açai is becoming much more readily available. Look for it in the freezer section.

1 tablespoon natural almond butter

1 cup plain whole milk Greek yogurt*

½ cup frozen strawberries

½ cup frozen blueberries

½ packet frozen açai purée

1 (1-inch) piece fresh ginger, peeled and sliced

½ lemon, zested and juiced

¼ to ½ cup unsweetened almond milk

1 teaspoon granulated monk fruit sweetener, optional

*You may substitute any nondairy yogurt, which would make this recipe vegan.

Suggested garnish:

½ tablespoon ground flaxseed

½ tablespoon chia seeds

1 tablespoon sliced almonds

½ cup fresh blueberries

½ cup fresh sliced strawberries

Place the almond butter, yogurt, frozen strawberries, blueberries, açai, ginger, lemon juice and zest, almond milk, and monk fruit sweetener in a blender and purée until well blended. Pour into a bowl.

Garnish with your favorite fruits, seeds, and nuts and enjoy.

Yogurt Flax Pancakes with Raspberry Compote

Serves 1
Active time: 10 minutes
Total time: 20 minutes

Jade and Sapphire
Emerald and Ruby (replace compote with fresh berries)

A delicious pancake made with flaxseeds, which are considered a superfood, high in fiber and omega-3 fatty acids. This recipe comes together quickly and can be doubled or tripled easily to serve a family. Make the compote ahead and keep warm. Serve with a side of fresh berries. You can also serve with the blueberry compote on page 243.

Pancake:

¼ cup whole-milk Greek yogurt*

½ teaspoon granulated monk fruit sweetener

¼ teaspoon cinnamon

2 large eggs

1¼ teaspoons ground flaxseeds

½ teaspoon baking powder

½ teaspoon vanilla extract

Pinch kosher salt

1 teaspoon butter

*You may substitute nondairy yogurt.

In a small bowl, combine the yogurt, monk fruit sweetener, cinnamon, eggs, flaxseeds, baking powder, vanilla extract, and salt and mix well.

Melt the butter in a small nonstick skillet over medium heat and add the pancake batter, smoothing it with the back of a spoon into a round pancake. Reduce the heat to low and cover the pan with a lid. Allow to cook until golden brown on the bottom, about 4 to 5 minutes. Slide the pancake onto a small plate and flip the uncooked side facedown into the skillet. Cook another 3 to 4 minutes until golden brown and cooked through. Serve with compote.

Compote:

½ cup raspberries, fresh or frozen

1 lemon, juiced

1 teaspoon granulated monk fruit sweetener

1 teaspoon pure vanilla extract

Combine the raspberries, lemon juice, monk fruit sweetener, and vanilla extract in a small saucepan. Mash the berries with a potato masher or the back of a wooden spoon. Cook over low heat until the berries break down slightly and the mixture thickens, 3 to 4 minutes.

SOUPS

Classic Vegetable Minestrone Soup

Serves 6, yields about 9 cups
Active time: 20 minutes
Total time: 50 minutes

Jade, Sapphire, Emerald, and Ruby

Hearty minestrone soup is a mainstay of Italian cuisine and varies from region to region. This version uses the rind from Parmigiano cheese, which infuses flavor into the broth. Next time you are left with a rind, simply rinse it, dry it, place it in a plastic bag, and freeze until you are ready to use. This version omits the traditional pasta but can be enjoyed with pure lentil pasta.

2 teaspoons extra-virgin olive oil

3 medium carrots, peeled and thinly sliced (¾ cup)

3 celery ribs, thinly sliced

1 large yellow onion, diced (2½ cups)

3 cloves garlic, minced

2 teaspoons dried Italian seasoning

1 (15-ounce) can cannellini beans, drained and rinsed

4 cups low-sodium chicken stock (or vegetable or beef stock)

1 (8-ounce) can tomato sauce

1 Parmigiano rind (optional)

2 medium zucchini, quartered lengthwise and sliced crosswise (1 pound 2 ounces)

5 ounces fresh baby spinach

¼ cup fresh basil, chopped to garnish

Grated Parmigiano, optional, to serve (suggest 2 tablespoons per serving)

Kosher salt, to taste

Ground black pepper, to taste

Preheat a large pot or Dutch oven over medium-high heat with the olive oil. Add the carrots, celery, onion, and garlic and cook until softened, 5 to 6 minutes. Season with salt and pepper and the Italian seasoning.

Add the beans, chicken stock, tomato sauce, and Parmigiano rind, if using. Season with salt and pepper. Bring to a boil and reduce to a simmer. Allow to simmer for 15 minutes, stirring occasionally. Add the zucchini and simmer again for 10 minutes or until the zucchini is tender. Remove from the heat, stir in the fresh spinach until it wilts. Taste for any seasoning.

Remove and discard the Parmigiano rind. Serve the soup in bowls and garnish with fresh basil and Parmigiano.

Can be refrigerated for 5 days or frozen in individual portions for up to 3 months.

Note: Omitting the Parmigiano and using vegetable broth makes this recipe suitable for vegans.

Chilled Avocado Soup

Serves 6, yields 6 cups
Active time: 10 minutes
Chill time: 4 hours

Jade, Sapphire, Emerald, and Ruby

This soup is light and refreshing, and it is lovely as an appetizer or a lunch or dinner entrée served with a skewer of grilled or poached shrimp. If you pick up an avocado and place it in the palm of your hand and squeeze gently without using your fingertips, and the avocado yields to gentle pressure, it's ripe and ready to use.

2 perfectly ripe avocados, pitted and peeled

4 cups low-sodium chicken broth

¼ cup roughly chopped shallot

Juice of 2 lemons, plus additional for seasoning

½ bunch cilantro leaves and stems, thoroughly rinsed and dried, plus
   additional for seasoning and garnish (about 1 cup packed stems and
   leaves)

Pinch cayenne pepper, optional

Kosher salt, to taste

Crème fraîche, sour cream, or olive oil

Combine the avocados, chicken broth, shallot, lemon juice, cilantro, and cayenne in a blender and purée until very smooth. Adjust seasoning to taste with salt and additional lemon juice and cilantro.

Refrigerate for at least 4 hours and serve very cold, with a dollop of crème fraîche or sour cream or a drizzle of olive oil. Garnish with a few cilantro leaves.

French Lentil Soup

Serves 6, yields 5 cups
Active time: 20 minutes
Total time: 50 minutes

Jade, Sapphire, Emerald, and Ruby

There's no other way to describe it: lentil soup is a hearty bowl of comfort. This version uses store-bought mirepoix, which significantly reduces prep time and supplies an amazingly creamy texture without using any cream. The trick is to purée a portion of the lentils once they are tender and then add them back in. You must use dried lentils to make this soup. There are many varieties—brown, green, red, and yellow. Brown lentils were used in this recipe, but feel free to experiment and find the type you like best.

2 tablespoons extra-virgin olive oil

Store-bought mirepoix containing about 1 cup each of chopped celery, onion, and carrot (or you can make your own)

2 teaspoons chopped garlic

1 teaspoon dried thyme

1 teaspoon dried rosemary

1¼ cups dried brown lentils

4 cups vegetable broth (or chicken broth); if you use vegetable broth, this recipe is suitable for vegans

1 (15-ounce) can diced tomatoes

1 to 1½ cups water

Kosher salt, to taste

Ground black pepper, to taste

Add the olive oil to a large heavy-bottomed pot or Dutch oven over medium heat. Add the mirepoix and garlic and sauté until the vegetables are soft, about 6 to 8 minutes, stirring occasionally, making sure they don't burn. Add the thyme and rosemary during the last minute of cooking and season with salt and pepper.

Add the lentils, broth, tomatoes, and water and bring the mixture to a boil. Season with salt and pepper. Reduce the heat and simmer for about 30 minutes, or until the lentils are tender.

Remove about 2 cups of the soup to a blender and process until smooth. Return the puréed lentils to the saucepan and stir to combine. Season to taste with salt and pepper and serve.

Refrigerate the leftovers for up to 7 days or freeze in individual portions for up to 3 months.

Gazpacho

Serves 6, yields 4 cups
Active time: 20 minutes
Chill time: 4 hours

Jade, Sapphire, Emerald, and Ruby

Gazpacho, a cold soup popular in Spain and Portugal, is made of raw blended vegetables. It is very refreshing, and a large bowl can be topped with grilled shrimp or chicken for a satisfying entrée. For a party, pour the gazpacho into a crystal pitcher and serve in shot glasses for a fun appetizer. It is versatile and delicious.

1 small red or white onion

2 pounds ripe tomatoes, plum or on the vine

½ red bell pepper, stemmed and seeded

1 English cucumber (12 ounces)

2 cloves garlic

2 teaspoons sherry vinegar

1 lemon, juiced

2 teaspoons kosher salt, plus additional to taste

¼ cup extra-virgin olive oil, plus more as needed

Roughly chop the tomatoes, pepper, cucumber, and onion. Add to a blender along with the garlic. Blend until quite smooth, scraping the sides of the blender as necessary. With the motor running, add the sherry vinegar, lemon juice, and about 2 teaspoons of kosher salt.

Slowly drizzle in the olive oil and allow to emulsify the way a salad dressing does. Continue to add olive oil until the desired consistency is reached. Refrigerate the gazpacho until very cold, at least 4 hours.

Adjust the salt and vinegar, to taste, before serving. If the soup is too thick, add some ice water.

To serve, drizzle with additional olive oil, if desired.

Spicy Slow-Cooked Black Bean Soup

Serves 8

Active time: 15 minutes

Total time: Overnight soak and 6 to 8 hours in slow cooker

Jade, Sapphire, Emerald, and Ruby

This incredibly simple-to-make soup is packed with protein and healthy ingredients, and if you choose your garnishes carefully, it is also naturally vegetarian, vegan, and gluten-free. It requires very little preparation: a slow cooker does all the work while you are away and will even keep it warm until you get home. You do have to think a day ahead to soak the beans overnight, but it's definitely worth the effort. If you don't like very spicy food, omit the jalapeños. For a soup that is a little bit spicier, don't remove the jalapeño seeds and add some sliced jalapeños as a garnish. It is a soup that can be enjoyed by all.

1 pound dried black beans, picked over for stones, rinsed and soaked overnight

1 red bell pepper, stemmed, seeded, and diced

2 jalapeño peppers, seeded and diced

½ large red onion, diced (about 1½ cups)

2 cloves garlic, minced

Chili powder (optional, as desired)

1 tablespoon ground cumin

1 teaspoon smoked paprika

1 teaspoon garlic powder

2 teaspoons kosher salt

4 cups low-sodium vegetable broth

1½ cups water

Garnishes:

1 fresh lime, cut in wedges

Sour cream

Shredded cheese (Mexican blend or Monterey Jack)

Roasted red peppers, diced

Chopped red onion

Avocado

Drain and rinse the soaked beans and add to a 6-quart slow cooker, along with the red pepper, jalapeños, onion, garlic, chili powder, cumin, smoked paprika, garlic powder, salt, vegetable broth, and water. Cook on high for 6 hours or low for 8 hours, until the flavors have blended and the soup has thickened nicely. Gently mash some of the black beans, using a potato masher, leaving the majority of the beans whole. Stir to combine and adjust any seasonings.

Serve with a squeeze of fresh lime and your choice of garnishes.

Can be refrigerated for 7 days or frozen in individual portions for up to 3 months.

Zucchini Curry Bisque

Serves 6
Active time: 25 minutes
Total time: 1 hour

Jade, Sapphire, Emerald, and Ruby

This quick and easy soup gets a little kick from the curry powder. It is a delicious everyday soup, but also perfect for company. For a light lunch, pair it with Herb-Roasted Spaghetti Squash (page 286) drizzled with olive oil and sprinkled with crumbled feta cheese.

Note: To make this a vegan recipe, use olive oil instead of butter and vegetable broth or water instead of chicken broth.

3 leeks or 1 large yellow onion

2 tablespoons extra-virgin olive oil

2 tablespoons unsalted butter or 2 additional tablespoons extra-virgin
  olive oil

2 teaspoons curry powder

5 to 6 zucchini (about 2 pounds), trimmed and sliced

3 cups low-sodium chicken broth, vegetable broth, or water

Kosher salt, to taste

Ground black pepper, to taste

¼ cup unsweetened almond milk

2 tablespoons unsalted butter, optional

2 tablespoons fresh lemon juice

Discard the top dark green portion of the leeks. Cut the remaining light green and white part of the leeks in half vertically. Rinse under cold water to clean and remove any grit. Thinly slice into half-moons. Or, if not using leeks, thinly slice the onion.

Heat the olive oil and butter (if using) in a large pot over medium heat. Add the leeks (or onions) and curry powder and sauté for about 5 minutes, stirring often. Add the zucchini and continue to cook until the vegetables are soft, another 5 to 7 minutes. Add the chicken broth. Bring to a boil, then reduce the heat and simmer for 20 minutes. Add additional water if the soup is too thick. Season with salt and pepper.

Allow the soup to cool slightly, about 5 minutes. Purée the soup with an immersion blender or in a high-speed blender until it is smooth and velvety. If it is too thick, thin with additional water or stock. Stir in the almond milk and additional butter until melted and combined. Stir in the lemon juice and season with salt and pepper as necessary and serve. Leftovers will keep in the fridge for up to 5 days.

SALADS

Deviled Eggs over Baby Spinach with Green Goddess Dressing

2 servings
Active time: 20 minutes
Total time: 30 minutes

Jade, Sapphire, Emerald, and Ruby

Named after a seasoning technique introduced by an Englishman, William Underwood, who launched his condiment and seasoning store in the Russian Wharf in Boston in 1822, this recipe is reinterpreted here with fresh, healthy ingredients.

Deviled Eggs:

4 large eggs
3 tablespoons mayonnaise
1 teaspoon mustard
Kosher salt, to taste
Ground black pepper, to taste
Paprika, to garnish

Cover the eggs with cold water in a medium saucepan. Prepare an ice bath. Bring the pan to a boil. Once boiling, shut off the heat, place the lid on the pot, and allow the eggs to sit in the hot water for 11 minutes. Immediately place the eggs in the ice water. Once they are cool, peel and remove the shells.

Carefully slice the eggs in half lengthwise. Remove the yolks to a bowl and set the whites aside. Mash the yolks thoroughly, add the mayonnaise and mustard, and stir until smooth. Season with salt and pepper. Place the yolk mixture into a zip-top bag and snip the corner with scissors. Pipe the filling into the center of each egg white. Set aside.

Green Goddess Dressing (yields ¾ cup):

½ cup parsley

½ cup baby spinach

1 tablespoon fresh tarragon

2 tablespoons fresh chives

1 clove garlic

1 anchovy fillet (optional)

1 lemon, juiced

2 teaspoons sherry vinegar

¼ cup grapeseed oil

¼ cup mayonnaise

Kosher salt, to taste

Ground black pepper, to taste

Combine the parsley, spinach, chives, tarragon, garlic, anchovy (if using), lemon juice, grapeseed oil, and sherry vinegar in a high-speed blender and blend until smooth. Add the mayonnaise and blend again. Season with salt and pepper.

To assemble:

4 cups baby spinach

Toss the baby spinach with desired amount of dressing. Set 4 deviled egg halves on top. Sprinkle with paprika.

Lemony Zucchini Salad

Serves 4, yields 5 cups
Active time: 15 minutes
Total time: 15 minutes

Jade, Sapphire, Emerald, and Ruby

This light, refreshing salad is a perfect starter or side dish any time of year, but especially in the summer. It doubles, triples, or quadruples easily to make a big bowl for a party. And because it doesn't require any cooking, it's a snap to prepare and there's no cleanup. It is certain to become one of your favorites. The recipe calls for one green zucchini and one yellow, but you can use the same color if that is all that is available.

1 green zucchini
1 yellow zucchini
¼ cup extra-virgin olive oil
Juice of 2 lemons, plus zest of 1 lemon
¼ cup torn fresh basil leaves
¼ cup torn fresh mint leaves or tarragon leaves
¼ cup grated Parmigiano
Kosher salt, to taste
Ground black pepper, to taste

Wash the zucchini and dry with paper towels. Slice them into ribbons using a carrot peeler. Stop when you get to the core with seeds. Try to avoid the seeds. Place the zucchini ribbons in a bowl and add the olive oil, lemon juice, lemon zest, basil, mint, Parmigiano, salt, and pepper and toss well to combine. Taste and adjust the seasonings if necessary.

Curry Chicken Salad in Lettuce Cups

Serves 2
Active time: 10 minutes
Total time: 30 minutes

Jade, Sapphire, Emerald, and Ruby

When you hear curry, it brings to mind an Indian dish, full of flavor and richness. This medley of spices can be used for vegetables or proteins and can be spicy or mild. In this dish, store-bought curry powder is used to create a chicken salad that is flavorful, easy to prepare, and can be served chilled or at room temperature.

1 boneless, skinless chicken breast (about 12 ounces)

1 small yellow onion, peeled and quartered

1 bay leaf

10 peppercorns

Dressing:

2 teaspoons grapeseed oil

2 tablespoons chopped yellow onion

2 tablespoons finely diced red bell pepper, pulp and seeds removed

4 teaspoons curry powder

¼ cup mayonnaise

2 teaspoons freshly squeezed lime juice

¼ cup peeled and chopped Granny Smith apple

1 stalk celery, chopped

2 tablespoons chopped fresh cilantro

2 tablespoons chopped fresh mint leaves

2 tablespoons roasted, unsalted peanuts, chopped (optional)

Kosher salt, to taste

Ground black pepper, to taste

Bibb or romaine lettuce leaves

Place the chicken breast in a saucepan with water to cover. Add the onion, bay leaf, and peppercorns. Bring to a boil over high heat, reduce to a simmer, cover, and cook 12 to 14 minutes until the chicken is completely cooked through. Remove the chicken from the poaching liquid, cool for 5 minutes, and shred using two forks.

Heat the grapeseed oil over medium heat in a medium skillet until shimmering. Add the onion and bell pepper and sauté until golden, about 3 minutes. Add the curry powder and cook for 1 minute, stirring constantly. Remove from the heat and place in a large bowl to cool. Add the mayonnaise, lime juice, apple, celery, cilantro, and mint to the large bowl and stir to combine. Add the chicken and stir to lightly coat. Season to taste with salt and pepper.

Spoon the chicken salad into individual lettuce leaves and top with chopped peanuts if desired.

Pasta Salad with Avocado and Chicken

Serves 3
Active time: 20 minutes
Total time: 40 minutes

Jade, Sapphire, Emerald, and Ruby
(only use pasta made with 100 percent lentils)

This beautiful, colorful salad made with red lentil pasta is full of healthy proteins, vegetables, and fats, and topped with a light, lemony dressing, it is a complete meal. You can do most of the preparation ahead of time. Cook the pasta right before serving, and the dish will be ready in about 20 minutes.

Red lentil pasta is high in protein and fiber and is, of course, gluten-free. The main benefit is that the carbohydrates will be absorbed more slowly due to the high fiber content, having a much more positive impact on blood sugar.

Poached Chicken:

1 boneless, skinless chicken breast (about 12 ounces)

1 small yellow onion, peeled and quartered

1 bay leaf

10 peppercorns

Place the chicken breast in a saucepan with water to cover. Add the onion, bay leaf, and peppercorns. Bring to a boil, reduce to a simmer, cover, and cook 12 to 14 minutes until completely cooked through. Remove the chicken from the poaching liquid, allow to cool for 5 minutes, and dice into ½-inch pieces.

For the Pasta Salad:

12 ounces red lentil pasta (made with 100 percent red lentil flour)

1 cup black or Kalamata olives, pitted and chopped

1 avocado, diced

20 grape tomatoes, halved

½ cup feta cheese, crumbled

5 ounces baby spinach

Lemon wedges, to serve

Bring a large pot of salted water to a boil. Cook the pasta according to the package directions. Begin checking the pasta earlier than usual to make sure it's tender with some bite and not overcooked. Drain it and rinse it under cold water to cool. Place the pasta in a large bowl.

For the Dressing:

¼ cup extra-virgin olive oil

1 teaspoon lemon zest

2 tablespoons fresh squeezed lemon juice

½ teaspoon kosher salt

Ground black pepper, to taste

Combine the olive oil, lemon zest, lemon juice, salt, and pepper in a mason jar or small sealed container and shake vigorously. Taste and adjust seasonings.

To assemble:

To the large bowl with the pasta, add the chicken, olives, avocado, and tomatoes. Add the dressing and toss lightly. Taste and adjust seasonings. Top with the crumbled feta cheese and serve over a bed of baby spinach with lemon wedges.

Smoked Salmon Rollups over Mixed Baby Greens

Serves 2 for lunch, 4 as an appetizer
Active time: 20 minutes
Total time: 20 minutes

Jade, Sapphire, Emerald, and Ruby

This flavorful dish can be easily doubled or tripled to serve for a light brunch or lunch, and it pairs nicely with Chilled Avocado Soup (see page 251). If you are fortunate enough to have a seafood counter where they can slice the salmon to order, that is great. If not, supermarkets carry packaged salmon in the deli section. Whipped cream cheese really works best in this recipe because it is much more spreadable than the block.

1 tablespoon capers, drained, rinsed, and chopped
1 tablespoon chopped red onion
1 tablespoon chopped fresh dill, plus additional to garnish
½ cup whipped cream cheese
8 thin slices smoked salmon (about ½ pound)
4 cups mixed baby greens
Lemon wedges, to serve
Ground black pepper, to taste

Combine the capers, red onion, dill, and cream cheese in a medium bowl. Season with pepper and mix to combine. Spoon 1 slightly rounded tablespoon of the cream cheese mixture onto each slice of salmon and roll it up. You should have 8 rolls.

To assemble, toss the baby greens with the dressing. Serve 2 or 4 roll-ups over baby greens, garnished with a squeeze of fresh lemon and a sprinkle of chopped dill.

Dressing:

¼ cup extra-virgin olive oil

2 tablespoons freshly squeezed lemon juice

1 clove garlic, minced

½ teaspoon kosher salt

Ground black pepper, to taste

Combine the olive oil, lemon juice, garlic, salt, and pepper in a mason jar or small sealed container and shake vigorously to blend well. Taste and adjust seasonings.

ENTRÉES

Whole Roasted Cauliflower with Herb Sauce

Serves 6

Active time: 15 minutes

Total time: 1 hour 15 minutes

Jade, Sapphire, Emerald, and Ruby

A whole roasted cauliflower is delicious and can be the centerpiece of your dining table, especially if you roast it in a pretty pie plate. It is also very versatile, and you can make use of whatever spices and herbs you have on hand. This recipe uses garam masala. But if you like herbs of Provence, you can sprinkle that on the cauliflower before roasting and maybe make a sauce with parsley and shallots to complement it. Feel free to experiment with the spice blends and herbs you enjoy. The cauliflower is the perfect vegetable for that.

Roasted Cauliflower:

1 medium whole cauliflower, 1½–2 lbs., leaves removed and core trimmed

2 tablespoons extra-virgin olive oil

5 teaspoons curry powder

1 to 2 tablespoons water

Pinch cayenne pepper (optional)

Kosher salt, to taste

Ground black pepper, to taste

Pure olive oil cooking spray, for greasing

Bring a large pot of salted water to a boil. Add the head of cauliflower and allow it to parboil for 10 to 15 minutes, just to cook slightly. Remove it from the pot and pat very dry with paper towels.

Preheat the oven to 400°F. Line a rimmed baking sheet with foil and grease it with olive oil cooking spray.

Place the cauliflower on the baking sheet. In a small bowl combine the olive oil, curry powder, water, and cayenne pepper, if using. Spread the mixture all over the head of cauliflower and season with salt and pepper. Tent the cauliflower with foil and roast for 35 to 40 minutes until almost tender when pierced with a paring knife. Remove the foil and return to the oven for another 10 to 20 minutes until golden brown and tender (keep checking the tenderness using a paring knife; if you like your cauliflower with some bite, roast for less time, or for very tender cauliflower, roast for more time).

Allow the cauliflower to cool for 5 to 10 minutes. Slice into wedges and serve with the herb sauce.

Herb Sauce:

1 clove garlic, grated

¼ cup chopped fresh basil

2 tablespoons chopped fresh mint leaves

1 tablespoon capers, drained, rinsed, and chopped

½ teaspoon red pepper flakes (optional)

¼ cup extra-virgin olive oil

2 tablespoons fresh lime juice

Kosher salt, to taste

Ground black pepper, to taste

Combine the garlic, basil, mint, capers, red pepper flakes, olive oil, and lime juice in a small bowl. Season with salt and pepper and set aside.

Grilled Shrimp Piccata

Serves 2
Active time: 10 minutes
Total time: 15 minutes

Jade, Sapphire, Emerald, and Ruby

Piccata is a classic Italian sauce made many different ways, depending on the chef. Some use garlic or shallots and white wine, and typically you will find it on veal or chicken. Here is a refreshing version made with lemon juice and capers for a quick shrimp dish that can be served over prepared millet or a side of lightly dressed greens for a delicious light meal.

Grilled Shrimp:

1 tablespoon extra-virgin olive oil
1 pound large shrimp, cleaned and deveined, tails on
Kosher salt, to taste
Ground black pepper, to taste

Preheat a grill or grill pan to medium-high heat. Toss the olive oil and shrimp in a large bowl and season with salt and pepper. Grill the shrimp for 2 to 3 minutes on each side until pink, opaque, and cooked through.

Piccata Sauce:

1 tablespoon extra-virgin olive oil
¼ cup finely chopped shallot
2 cloves garlic, minced
¼ cup fresh lemon juice, plus ½ teaspoon lemon zest
1 tablespoon capers, drained and rinsed
½ cup low-sodium chicken stock
1 tablespoon unsalted butter
2 tablespoons chopped parsley
Kosher salt, to taste
Ground black pepper, to taste

Heat the olive oil in a medium skillet over medium-high heat. Add the shallot and garlic and cook until softened, 2 to 3 minutes. Add the lemon zest, juice, capers, and chicken stock. Bring to a boil and reduce to a simmer. Allow to simmer for 3 to 5 minutes or until the mixture has reduced by half. Season with salt and pepper.

Remove from the heat and whisk in the butter until melted. Stir in the parsley and season again, to taste, as needed. Toss the grilled shrimp in the warm sauce and serve.

Pan-Roasted Salmon with Dill

Serves 2
Active time: 10 minutes
Total time: 15 minutes

Jade, Sapphire, Emerald, and Ruby

This is a simple but delicious preparation for salmon. Easy enough for every day, and elegant enough for a dinner party when served over Cauliflower Purée (page 282) or with Haricots Verts with Mushrooms and Shallots (page 283). Buy the freshest fish you can find. If that is not an option in your area, online purveyors sell quality fish that is frozen very soon after it is caught, and they have the highest standards. This recipe can easily be prepared for one, or the second fillet makes a delicious salad the next day, shredded over greens, drizzled with olive oil and lemon juice.

1 tablespoon extra-virgin olive oil

2 (6-ounce) wild salmon fillets, skin removed

¼ cup unsalted butter

2 tablespoons fresh lemon juice

¼ cup chopped fresh dill

2 tablespoons chopped fresh parsley

Kosher salt, to taste

Ground black pepper, to taste

Heat a large nonstick sauté pan over medium-high heat with olive oil. Season the salmon fillets with salt and pepper.

Add the salmon, top side down, to the pan and allow to cook for 1 to 2 minutes. Flip the salmon fillets over and add the butter. Place a lid on the pan and allow to cook for 1 to 2 minutes or until the butter turns a light golden brown.

Add the lemon juice and place the lid back on the pan. Reduce the heat to medium and allow to cook for 6 to 9 minutes or until the salmon is the desired level of doneness (if the sauce reduces too much or looks like it may burn, add a few tablespoons of water).

Remove from the heat and stir in fresh dill and parsley. Season again with salt and pepper, if desired, and serve.

Chicken Cutlets with Shallots and Capers

Serves 4

Active time: 20 minutes

Total time: 35 minutes

Jade, Sapphire, Emerald, and Ruby

With ingredients that are easy to keep on hand and a preparation that is so very simple, this meal, made in one pan, is sure to become your weeknight go-to. It is delicious served over Cauliflower Purée (page 282) or with Haricots Verts with Mushrooms and Shallots (page 283). Or for an even lighter meal, serve alongside an arugula salad with a lemony dressing.

1 pound thin-sliced, boneless, skinless chicken breasts (about 4 to 5)

Kosher salt, to taste

Ground black pepper, to taste

½ cup almond flour

4 tablespoons unsalted butter, divided

2 tablespoons extra-virgin olive oil

1 shallot, thinly sliced

1 cup low-sodium chicken stock

1 cup dry white wine

2 tablespoons capers, rinsed

2 tablespoons chopped fresh parsley

Season the chicken liberally on both sides with salt and pepper and dredge in the almond flour. Set it aside on a rack.

Heat 2 tablespoons of the unsalted butter and the olive oil in a large sauté pan over medium heat. Add the chicken and sauté until golden, turning once, about 3 to 4 minutes per side. Remove it to a platter and keep warm.

Return the pan to medium heat and melt 1 tablespoon of the butter. Add the shallots and sauté until soft, about 5 minutes. Add the stock and wine and deglaze the pan, scraping up the brown bits with a wooden spoon. Bring to a boil and reduce by half, another 5 to 7 minutes. Season with salt and pepper.

Add the chicken and any collected juices back to the pan and simmer 3 to 5 minutes. Swirl in the remaining 1 tablespoon of butter, sprinkle with capers and parsley, and serve.

Spice-Rubbed Spatchcocked Chicken

Serves 4

Active time: 15

Total time: 1 hour 20 minutes

Jade, Sapphire, Emerald, and Ruby

Spatchcocking is a technique that entails removing the backbone of the chicken and flattening it, which exposes a greater amount of skin, allowing it to get crispy. It also yields a perfectly roasted chicken in a much shorter time than roasting the whole bird. In order to have evenly browned, crispy skin, whether you are cooking the whole bird or parts, the skin must be dry. The drier the skin, the crispier it will be. If you have the time to plan ahead and can wash and dry the chicken and refrigerate it overnight, it will ensure the crispiest skin. This rub works great on chicken parts and whole chickens as well.

1 3½- to 4-pound chicken, washed and patted dry, and preferably
    refrigerated uncovered overnight—to ensure an extra-crispy skin

1 teaspoon ground cumin

2 teaspoons onion powder

2 teaspoons garlic powder

1 tablespoon kosher salt

½ teaspoon dried oregano

½ teaspoon paprika

½ teaspoon ground black pepper

1 to 2 tablespoons harissa paste (depending on spice preference)

¼ cup extra-virgin olive oil

2 tablespoons chopped fresh mint leaves, to serve

Lemon wedges, to serve

Place the chicken, breast side down, on a cutting board, with the legs facing you. With very sharp kitchen shears, cut along one side of the backbone, then the other. Remove the bone and discard it or place it in a freezer bag to make stock in the future. Set the chicken aside at room temperature for 20 to 30 minutes.

Meanwhile, preheat the oven to 450°F. Line a rimmed baking sheet with foil.

Combine the cumin, onion powder, garlic powder, kosher salt, dried oregano, paprika, and black pepper in a small bowl. Add the harissa and olive oil and stir to form a paste.

Pat the chicken very dry on both sides with paper towels. Place the chicken breast side up and press on the breastbone to crack the sternum and flatten the breasts. Rub the spice paste over the chicken on both sides and under the skin, being careful not to tear the skin.

Place the chicken on the baking sheet. Roast the chicken for about 35 to 40 minutes. Check the thigh for doneness; the juices should run clear and a meat thermometer should register 165°F.

If you desire extra crispy skin, preheat the broiler. Place the chicken under the broiler for 2 to 6 minutes until skin is extra golden and crispy.

Allow the chicken to rest tented with foil for 15 minutes before carving. You can carve the chicken as you would a turkey: remove the legs and wings, and then remove the breasts from the bone and slice them. Serve garnished with fresh mint and lemon wedges.

Serve with Cauliflower Purée (page 282).

Garam Masala Lamb Chops

Serves 4–6

Active time: 18 minutes

Total time: 18 minutes, plus 2 hours 30 minutes marinating

Jade, Sapphire, Emerald, and Ruby

Lamb chops are the perfect special-occasion treat. Whether it's a romantic dinner, a wine club dinner party, or a summer barbecue, this recipe's got you covered. With simple ingredients in a make-ahead marinade prepared in a food processor, you will have plenty of time to get everything else ready for the evening ahead.

5–6 cloves garlic, roughly chopped

1 (1-inch) piece ginger root, peeled and coarsely chopped

½ medium white onion, coarsely chopped

2 tablespoons garam masala

Juice of 1 lemon

1 teaspoon kosher salt

Red chili flakes, to taste

2 racks of lamb, cut into individual chops (about 3 pounds, 16 lamb rib chops about ¾-inch thick)

2 tablespoons extra-virgin olive oil, plus additional as needed

2 tablespoons cilantro, chopped to garnish

Purée the garlic, ginger root, onion, garam masala, lemon juice, salt, and chili flakes in a blender or food processor until smooth. If the mixture is too thick, add some water.

Place the lamb chops in a bowl with a cover or sealable plastic bag, add the marinade, and mix thoroughly, making sure that the chops are completely covered by the marinade. Refrigerate for 2 hours.

Remove chops from refrigerator and bring them to room temperature for 30 minutes. Discard any excess marinade. Preheat a large cast iron skillet, grill, or grill pan over medium heat with the olive oil. Cook the chops until they reach the temperature of 145°F on a meat thermometer, 2 to 3 minutes per side for medium rare, turning once. This will have to be done in batches; add more olive oil if necessary. Set the chops aside on a plate and allow them to rest for 5 minutes before serving.

Garnish with chopped cilantro. Serve with Cauliflower Purée (page 282).

Note: This marinade is also delicious with chicken. Use the chicken parts you prefer. The marinade provides enough for 8 bone-in, skin-on thighs. Marinate the chicken overnight and then grill on an outdoor grill or bake in the oven at 450°F for 35 minutes. If you prefer boneless, skinless thighs, marinate for only about 20 minutes. They will cook very quickly on the grill or under the broiler, about 10 minutes, so watch them carefully.

Puerto Rican Pernil Pork Chops

Serves 2
Active time: 10 minutes
Total time: 60 minutes, plus 6 hours marinating up to overnight

Jade, Sapphire, Emerald, and Ruby

This marinade comes from a Latin American dish called *pernil*, which is a slow-roasted pork shoulder. It's marinated for many hours, then slow-roasted for many hours, and then cooked at a high temperature to crisp the skin. In everyday life, there isn't time for *pernil,* but there is time for these flavorful, juicy pork chops. With a little planning, an overnight marinade is best to really infuse the chops with flavor.

1 tablespoon chopped garlic (about 3 garlic cloves)

3 tablespoons plus 2 teaspoons extra-virgin olive oil, divided

1 tablespoon white wine vinegar

2 teaspoons dried oregano

½ teaspoon chili powder

¼ teaspoon ground cumin

Pinch cayenne pepper

1 teaspoon kosher salt

1 teaspoon ground black pepper

2 bone-in center cut pork chops, ¾- to 1-inch thick

Lime wedges, to serve

Combine the chopped garlic, 3 of the tablespoons olive oil, white wine vinegar, dried oregano, chili powder, cumin, cayenne, salt, and pepper in a mini food processor and process until smooth. If you don't have a mini food processor, whisk to combine and mash the chopped garlic, using the bottom of a drinking glass.

Rinse the pork chops and pat dry with a paper towel. Place them in a resealable plastic bag. Add the marinade ingredients. Seal the bag and massage the pork chops to make sure the marinade is evenly distributed. Refrigerate for at least 6 hours, or overnight.

Remove the pork chops from the refrigerator at least 30 minutes before cooking to bring them to room temperature. Discard the marinade.

Heat a large cast iron skillet over medium-high heat. Add the remaining 2 teaspoons olive oil and heat until shimmering. Add the pork chops and allow them to cook for 8 to 12 minutes, flipping halfway through, until both sides are golden brown and slightly crispy, and the internal temperature on a meat thermometer is 145°F. Remove the pork chops to a plate and allow them to rest for 5 to 10 minutes. Serve with lime wedges.

Spiced Lamb Ragu

Serves 4, yields 3 cups lamb sauce
Active time: 25 minutes
Total time: 45 minutes

Jade, Sapphire, Emerald, and Ruby

This meat sauce, typically made with ground lamb because of its delicate flavor, can also be made with ground chicken or turkey. The onion is soaked in water to soften it and remove some of the acidity. You can refrigerate any leftovers for 3 to 4 days. To reheat, place the sauce in a pan over low heat, add some water, and warm, stirring occasionally.

2 tablespoons extra-virgin olive oil

1 medium sweet onion, very finely diced (about 1 cup)

1 carrot, peeled and finely diced

1 rib celery, peeled and finely diced

2 cloves garlic, minced

2 teaspoons Italian seasoning

1 teaspoon ground coriander

½ teaspoon ground cinnamon

1 pound ground lamb

⅓ cup dry white wine

1 (28-ounce) can whole peeled tomatoes, crushed with hands

2 cups water

1 tablespoon unsalted butter

1 Herb-Roasted Spaghetti Squash (page 286) or 1 pound red lentil pasta
    prepared according to the package directions

Kosher salt, to taste

Ground black pepper, to taste

2 tablespoons grated Parmigiano Reggiano cheese, to garnish

Fresh basil leaves, to garnish

Heat the olive oil in a large heavy-bottomed pot or Dutch oven over medium-high heat. Add the onion, carrot, and celery and season with salt and pepper. Cook until the vegetables are tender and golden, 4 to 5 minutes. Add the garlic, Italian seasoning, coriander, and cinnamon, and cook an additional minute.

Add the ground lamb and sauté over medium heat, breaking up the meat with a wooden spoon, for about 10 to 12 minutes or until browned and cooked through. Season with salt and pepper.

Add the white wine, tomatoes, and water, bring to a boil, and reduce to a simmer. Season with salt and pepper. Allow to simmer until the sauce has thickened, 20 to 25 minutes. Remove from the heat and stir in the butter and additional black pepper, stirring constantly until well combined. Serve with spaghetti squash or pasta and toss to coat.

Garnish with grated Parmigiano Reggiano and fresh basil leaves.

Citrus Skirt Steak with Chimichurri

Active time: 25 minutes
Total time: 55 minutes

Jade, Sapphire, Emerald, and Ruby

Skirt steak is a long cut of beef that is one of the most flavorful, but it requires a little extra preparation. In this recipe, you prepare the steak by pounding it lightly with a meat tenderizer on both sides, then marinate the steak in citrus, which helps to break down the toughness of the meat. Once cooked, it's topped with chimichurri, which is a sauce used in South American and Mexican cuisine. It can be used both in cooking and as a condiment. It has many national variations. Experiment by using herbs and spices you like.

2 garlic cloves, finely minced

2 tablespoons chopped cilantro or parsley

1 teaspoon dried oregano

1 lemon, juiced

1 lime, juiced

2 tablespoons extra-virgin olive oil

1 teaspoon kosher salt

1 teaspoon ground black pepper

1½ pounds skirt steak, trimmed of excess fat, and lightly pounded on
    both sides with a meat tenderizer

Chimichurri (page 280)

Mix the garlic, cilantro or parsley, and oregano in a small bowl. Add lemon juice, lime juice, olive oil, salt, and pepper. Stir to combine.

Place the steak in a large zip-top bag and pour the marinade over the meat. Seal the bag and turn it over several times to make sure the steak is completely coated. Marinate at room temperature for 30 minutes.

Remove the steak from the bag and discard the marinade. Heat a large cast iron pan, grill, or grill pan over medium-high heat. Add the steak to the pan and cook to your desired temperature, approximately 2 to 3 minutes per side for medium rare, depending on the thickness of the steak.

Remove the steak to a cutting board, tent with foil, and let it stand for 10 minutes. Cut the steak diagonally against the grain into thin slices. Serve with Chimichurri (page 280).

Chimichurri:

1 to 2 bunches parsley leaves and stems, chopped (about 3/4 cup, chopped)

3 tablespoons chopped fresh mint leaves

1 jalapeño, seeded and finely diced

1 cup finely diced red onion

½ cup extra-virgin olive oil (or more, to taste)*

¼ cup red wine vinegar (or more, to taste)*

Kosher salt, to taste

Ground black pepper, to taste

Mix the parsley, mint, jalapeño, and red onion together in a small bowl. Add the olive oil and red wine vinegar and mix to make a loose sauce. Season with salt and pepper, to taste. Cover the bowl with plastic wrap and leave it on the counter for at least 2 hours for the flavors to meld. Any leftovers can be refrigerated for up to 1 week. Remove from the refrigerator 1 hour before serving to bring to room temperature.

*You can alter the measurements of the oil and vinegar to suit your taste and the consistency you like. You may also substitute freshly squeezed lemon juice for the vinegar.

ACCOMPANIMENTS/SIDES

Aglio e Olio

Serves: 4, yields 3½ cups using spaghetti squash
Active time: 10 minutes
Total time: 10 minutes

Jade, Sapphire, Emerald, and Ruby

The translation of *aglio e olio* is garlic and oil. It is a very traditional pasta dish from Naples, and extremely popular because the sauce is prepared with very simple ingredients that most people have on hand. The dish comes together very quickly while the pasta, usually spaghetti, is cooking. Although called garlic and oil, this recipe includes some other ingredients for a much more flavorful dish.

¼ cup extra-virgin olive oil

½ medium yellow onion, finely chopped (about ⅓ cup)

2 garlic cloves, minced

2 tablespoons fresh parsley leaves, finely chopped, plus additional to
    garnish

1 teaspoon dried oregano

Pinch red pepper flakes (optional)

Kosher salt, to taste

Ground black pepper, to taste

1 Herb-Roasted Spaghetti Squash (page 286) or 1 pound red lentil pasta
    prepared according to package directions (3½ cups cooked spaghetti
    squash)

Boiling water, if needed

¼ cup grated Parmigiano Reggiano

Heat the olive oil in a sauté pan over medium heat. Add the onion and sauté until soft and golden, about 4 to 5 minutes. Reduce the heat to low, add the garlic, and sauté for an additional minute, being careful not to let it burn. Add the parsley, oregano, and red pepper flakes, if using, and season with salt and pepper.

Add the prepared herb-roasted spaghetti squash or red lentil pasta to the garlic and oil mixture and stir to combine, allowing the sauce to be absorbed. Add 1 to 2 tablespoons of boiling water to loosen the mixture, if necessary.

Sprinkle with the Parmigiano Reggiano and additional parsley and serve.

Cauliflower Purée

Serves 4, yields 1 cup
Active time: 10 minutes
Total time: 15 minutes

Jade, Sapphire, Emerald, and Ruby

This creamy, buttery purée makes a delicious alternative to mashed potatoes. Cauliflower florets in microwaveable bags are widely available in supermarkets and make preparing this dish a snap. Serve it with Spice-Rubbed Spatchcocked Chicken (page 272) or Chicken Cutlets with Shallots and Capers (page 270).

1 (10-ounce) bag of cauliflower florets or one whole medium-sized
    cauliflower
3 tablespoons unsalted butter, softened
Kosher salt, to taste
Ground black pepper, to taste

Bring a small pot of salted water to a boil. Add the cauliflower and cook until very tender, 7 to 9 minutes. Drain. Alternatively, microwave the cauliflower according to package directions.

Add the cooked cauliflower to the bowl of a food processor fitted with the blade attachment and purée until very smooth. Add the butter and process until it is incorporated.

Season to taste with salt and pepper, and keep warm until ready to serve.

Haricots Verts with Mushrooms and Shallots

Serves 4
Active time: 15 minutes
Total time: 25 minutes

Jade, Sapphire, Emerald, and Ruby

This dish, reminiscent of the old-school string bean casserole served at Thanksgiving, has been elevated by using haricots verts, baby bella mushrooms, and shallots. With haricots verts in microwaveable bags now readily available in supermarkets, preparing this delicious side dish is very quick and easy.

8 ounces haricots verts in a microwaveable bag or 8 ounces trimmed
    string beans*
3 tablespoons unsalted butter
2 shallots, thinly sliced
1 (8-ounce) container baby bella mushrooms or other mushrooms, wiped
    clean and sliced
2 tablespoons water
¼ cup low-sodium chicken broth or vegetable broth
¼ cup unsweetened almond milk
Kosher salt, to taste
Freshly ground black pepper, to taste
Sliced almonds, optional

Bring a medium pot of salted water to a light boil. Add the haricots verts and cook for 6 to 7 minutes or until crisp tender. Drain and rinse under cold water. Alternatively, microwave following the package instructions. Slice the slightly cooled haricots verts into thirds and set aside.

Melt the butter in a large sauté pan. Add the shallots and sauté over medium heat until soft, about 3 minutes. Add the mushrooms and cook, stirring, for 6 to 7 minutes, until soft and golden brown. After the mushrooms have been cooking for 1 to 2 minutes, add 2 tablespoons of water and season with salt and pepper, to taste.

Once the mushrooms are tender, add the chicken broth, bring to a boil, and season to taste with salt and pepper. Reduce the heat to low and add the haricots verts and simmer for 3 minutes. Add the almond milk, adjust the seasonings, toss, sprinkle with sliced almonds if using, and serve.

Note: If you don't like using a microwave, or can't find haricots verts, no problem. Just trim string beans and blanch them in salted boiling water for 6 to 7 minutes, then drain them and proceed with the recipe.

Pinto Beans Sofrito

Serves 4
Active time: 5 minutes
Total time: 15 minutes

Jade, Sapphire, Emerald, and Ruby

Beans are a staple in every Latin American cuisine, as well as on the MetaKura meal plan. Black beans, kidney beans, pink beans, and pinto beans are a few bean varieties. Beans are tasty and a really healthy protein choice. This recipe for pinto beans uses sofrito, which is a tomato base. If you can't find it, or are inspired, there is a recipe following.

2 tablespoons extra-virgin olive oil

¼ cup sofrito (Homemade Sofrito, page 286)

1 tablespoon tomato paste

1 teaspoon ground turmeric

½ teaspoon ground cumin

Pinch cayenne pepper, optional

1 cup low-sodium chicken stock or vegetable stock

1 (16-ounce) can pinto beans, drained and rinsed

½ lime, zested and juiced

Kosher salt, to taste

Ground black pepper, to taste

Warm the olive oil in a small saucepan over medium heat. Add the sofrito and cook until softened, 1 to 2 minutes. Add the tomato paste, turmeric, cumin, and cayenne, if using, and cook to caramelize the tomato paste and toast the spice, 1 minute or so. Add the chicken stock and beans, and stir to combine. Season with salt and pepper. Bring to a boil, then reduce the heat to medium-low and simmer for 8 to 10 minutes, until the sauce has thickened and the beans are tender. Stir in the lime zest and juice and serve.

Homemade Sofrito

Makes 1¼ cups

Active time: 10 minutes

Total time: 15 minutes

Jade, Sapphire, Emerald, and Ruby

1 small yellow onion, roughly chopped

3 garlic cloves, roughly chopped

2 green peppers (such as a Cubanelle, banana, or Anaheim), stemmed, seeded, and roughly chopped

5 plum tomatoes, seeded and roughly chopped (1 pound 2 ounces)

¼ cup extra-virgin olive oil

1 teaspoon paprika

Kosher salt, to taste

Ground black pepper, to taste

To the bowl of a food processor fitted with the blade attachment, add the onion, garlic, green peppers, tomatoes, olive oil, and paprika. Pulse until finely chopped. Season with salt and pepper.

Herb-Roasted Spaghetti Squash

Serves: 2–4, yields 3½ cups

Active time: 5 minutes

Cooking time: 45 minutes–1 hour

Total time: 50–65 minutes

Jade, Sapphire, Emerald, and Ruby

Spaghetti squash are available in many different shapes and colors, with the yellow variety being the most common. The center has many large seeds, and it looks similar to other types of winter squash when raw, but when it is cooked, it comes away in strands that resembles spaghetti, hence its name. It is ready to be served as a side dish, or as a substitute for pasta topped with your favorite sauce.

1 spaghetti squash (about 2½ pounds), cut in half lengthwise, seeds removed

2 tablespoons extra-virgin olive oil

1 teaspoon dried thyme

Kosher salt, to taste

Ground black pepper, to taste

Preheat the oven to 425°F. Line a baking sheet with parchment paper.

Drizzle each half of the squash with 1 tablespoon of olive oil, sprinkle with ½ teaspoon thyme, and season with salt and pepper. Place cut side down on the baking sheet. Bake for 45 minutes to 1 hour, until the squash is tender (you should be able to easily pierce it with the tip of a knife).

Allow the squash to cool until comfortable to touch. Using a fork, gently scrape the squash into long strands and remove them to a bowl.

It's ready to use as a substitute for pasta in a recipe, or sprinkle with cheese of your choice and fresh chopped herbs and serve as a side dish.

SAUCES

Puttanesca Sauce

Serves 4; makes 2¾ cups sauce
Active time: 20 minutes
Total time: 40 minutes

Jade, Sapphire, Emerald, and Ruby

There are various recipes and stories surrounding the name *puttanesca*, dating back to the early nineteenth century. Under its current name, it appeared in cookbooks in the 1960s. The general theme of the sauce is that it can be made quickly, in between other obligations, or clients, and so the allusion to the *puttana*, or prostitute. It's a slightly scandalous name for a fragrant and flavorful sauce that comes together quickly with pretty basic items you can keep on hand.

1 (28-ounce) can whole peeled Italian tomatoes
¼ cup extra-virgin olive oil
4 cloves garlic, peeled and minced
3 anchovy fillets, thoroughly mashed (or 2 teaspoons of anchovy paste)
Pinch red pepper flakes
1 tablespoon capers, drained
¼ cup olives, either oil-cured or Kalamata
10–12 fresh basil leaves
1½ cups water
Kosher salt, to taste
Ground black pepper, to taste
1 Herb-Roasted Spaghetti Squash (page 286) or 1 pound red lentil pasta
     prepared according to package directions
¼ cup Pecorino cheese, grated

Pour the Italian tomatoes into a bowl and crush with your hand. Set them aside.

Heat the olive oil over medium heat in a medium heavy-bottomed pot. Add the garlic, mashed anchovies or paste, and red pepper flakes. Cook, stirring from time to time, until the garlic is golden and the anchovies melt, making sure it doesn't burn, about 3 minutes. Add the tomatoes, capers, olives, and basil. Pour 1½ cups of water into the tomato can, then pour it into the sauce. Season with salt and pepper.

Bring the sauce to a boil and reduce the heat to a simmer. Cook, stirring occasionally, until the sauce is reduced and slightly thickened, 25 to 30 minutes. Season with additional salt and black pepper, if needed.

Add the prepared spaghetti squash or red lentil pasta to the sauce and toss to coat.

Serve with grated Pecorino cheese.

Quick Marinara Sauce

Serves 6 (makes 2½ cups)
Active time: 10 minutes
Total time: 25 minutes

Jade, Sapphire, Emerald, and Ruby

A really good recipe to have in your arsenal is a quick marinara sauce. You can have dinner ready in less than 30 minutes, because discounting the fresh basil, which is lovely to add but not necessary, you need only basic pantry items. Not only can you serve it over millet, red lentil pasta, or prepared Herb-Roasted Spaghetti Squash (page 286), but poaching eggs in tomato sauce is delicious—it even has a name—Eggs in Purgatory! Try it.

2 tablespoons extra-virgin olive oil

3 garlic cloves, finely minced

¼ cup finely chopped yellow onion

1 teaspoon dried thyme

¼ teaspoon red chili flakes

1 (28-ounce) can Italian whole peeled tomatoes, pureed in a blender just
    until smooth, about 10 seconds—do not overprocess

1 cup water

7–11 fresh basil leaves, if available (do not use dried)

Kosher salt, to taste

Ground black pepper, to taste

Heat the olive oil in a medium pot over medium heat until warm. Add
the garlic and onion and cook until softened, about 3 minutes. Add the
thyme and chili flakes and season with salt and pepper. Add the tomatoes and season again with salt and pepper.

Rinse the tomato can with 1 cup of water and pour it into the pot.
Bring to a boil and reduce to a simmer. Allow the sauce to simmer, stirring occasionally, for 15 minutes, until slightly thickened. Remove from
the heat and stir in the fresh basil leaves. Season again as needed.

The sauce can be refrigerated for 5 days or frozen for up to 3 months.

DESSERTS

Chocolate Ricotta Mousse

Serves 2, yields 1 cup
Active time: 15 minutes
Total time: 15 minutes

Jade, Sapphire, Emerald, and Ruby

This mousse is so creamy and delicious that it is sure to satisfy anyone's chocolate cravings. You can easily double or triple this recipe. For a dinner party, serve it in martini glasses or champagne coupes for an elegant presentation, and top with a tablespoon of Vanilla Sauce (page 294).

½ cup ricotta, whole milk or part skim

2 to 3 tablespoons unsweetened cocoa powder

½ teaspoon pure vanilla extract

2 tablespoons granulated monk fruit sweetener

1 egg white

⅛ teaspoon cream of tartar

Combine the ricotta, cocoa powder, vanilla extract, and monk fruit sweetener in the bowl of a food processor fitted with the blade attachment and mix until very smooth. Transfer to a bowl.

Place the egg white and cream of tartar in a small bowl. Using an electric mixer, beat until stiff peaks form. Fold the egg white into the ricotta mixture until it is completely blended.

Divide the mousse into two ramekins. Serve immediately or cover with plastic wrap and refrigerate until ready to serve.

Raspberry Ricotta Mousse

Serves 4
Active time: 15 minutes
Total time: 15 minutes

Jade, Sapphire, Emerald, and Ruby

This light, creamy dessert is so decadent, no one will ever know that you whipped it up in 15 minutes and used only five ingredients. Serve it in beautiful glass bowls garnished with dark chocolate curls for special guests.

> 1 cup ricotta, whole milk or part skim
> ¼ cup granulated monk fruit sweetener
> 1 cup fresh raspberries, plus more for garnish, if desired
> 1 teaspoon vanilla extract
> ⅓ cup heavy cream

Combine the ricotta, monk fruit sweetener, raspberries, and vanilla extract in a food processor. Blend until smooth and transfer to a bowl.

Pour the heavy cream into a medium bowl and beat with an electric hand mixer until it is thick and fluffy. Fold the whipped cream into the raspberry ricotta mixture until well combined. Spoon the mousse into 4 serving bowls. Cover with plastic wrap and refrigerate until ready to serve.

Garnish with fresh raspberries if desired.

Poached Pears with Vanilla Sauce

Serves 2
Active time: 35 minutes
Total time: 45 minutes

Jade (unrestricted)
Sapphire (once every two weeks)
Emerald and Ruby (use crunchy uncooked pear, as sugar
content increases with cooking)

This elegant dessert is the perfect ending to a special meal. The whole pears are poached in a lightly spiced liquid and chilled, and then served with a creamy vanilla sauce. It can easily be doubled or tripled and is the perfect make-ahead dessert for a dinner party. Garnish with a few dark chocolate curls for a spectacular presentation.

Pears:

¼ cup granulated monk fruit sweetener

5 cups water

2 vanilla beans, split lengthwise

3 cinnamon sticks

2 Bosc pears, cored and peeled (should be fairly underripe and crunchy)

Place the monk fruit sweetener, water, vanilla beans, and cinnamon sticks in a medium saucepan. Bring to a boil, reduce to a simmer, and add the pears. Cook for 15 to 20 minutes, until the pears are just tender.

Remove the pears from the poaching liquid and allow them to cool. They may be left at room temperature or covered with plastic wrap and refrigerated. Remove the cinnamon stick and vanilla bean and discard.

Boil the poaching liquid until it's reduced by half. Allow it to cool, then refrigerate until ready to use.

Vanilla Sauce:

3 tablespoons granulated monk fruit sweetener

1 tablespoon almond flour (not almond meal)

1 large egg

2 tablespoons unsalted butter

1¼ cups heavy cream

Pinch kosher salt

1 tablespoon vanilla extract

Combine the monk fruit sweetener, almond flour, egg, butter, heavy cream, and salt in a small saucepan. Cook over low heat, whisking constantly, until the butter melts and sauce thickens, about 10 minutes. Remove from heat, whisk in the vanilla, and allow it to cool completely. Refrigerate until ready to use.

To serve, place one pear in the center of a plate. Drizzle with 1 teaspoon of poaching liquid. Pour some vanilla sauce over the top of the pear and let it run down the sides. Spoon more sauce around the bottom of the pear.

You can access more recipes and food choices at www.metakura.com

EPILOGUE

In this, the post-Neolithic stage of our human metabolic evolution, we exercise less, we eat more, we sleep less, and we experience new types of stress than did our ancestors. Human endeavor has helped to make our food sources more secure. But we have done so through the over-processing of foods and drink to make their shelf lives longer. Today people all over the world may live longer, but we will likely be less metabolically robust and healthy than our forebearers. Those of us most at risk for medical calamities are those who by being insulin resistant are more genetically adapted to a prehistoric life. This segment of the population continues to grow.

However, we both believe that all over the world people are fighting back to reclaim their health, for their right to wholesome food, and to find quiet spaces in their lives. Most of all, people are acquiring the necessary knowledge to be articulate, well-informed champions of their own well-being. We applaud each and every one of you.

ACKNOWLEDGMENTS

Our greatest debt of gratitude is to our many patients, who have taught us most of what we know. Their beliefs and revelations continually serve to nudge us to reevaluate our knowledge. As well, we offer warm-hearted appreciation to the clinic patients who have permitted us to tell their medical stories, with protective measures to camouflage their identities.

This book was born after a series of exploratory conversations with a dear friend, the subtle yet masterful sculptor of ideas and editor, Carrie Thornton. We are immensely fortunate that as she got more acquainted with our work, she encouraged us to step outside the busy world of our clinic to share our expertise with new audiences.

We are indebted, too, for the vital support that we received from other quarters. Our agent Jaidree Braddix's depth of expertise and resourcefulness have been invaluable. Seema Mahanian, our editor at Hachette, has deftly steered the book for publication with energy and élan. Sheila Curry Oakes's and Rebecca Maines's consummate gifts for clarity enhance every page.

We also wish to especially honor the contributions of our Meta-Kura Clinic colleagues, whose years of dedication to our patients have made this book possible: Chiefly among them, we owe an immeasurable karmic debt to Luz Ricablanca. We also wish to express our gratitude to Morgan Howard, Sarah Marschany, and Matthew Wise. Blessed with Vivian Cioffi's generous gift of fresh and easy recipes, our ideas on nutrition have leaped to life in delicious incarnations.

Our book has benefited immensely from the insights of countless experts, most notably Dr. Gerald Reaven and Dr. Doug Coleman. Over the years, Dr. Derek LeRoith has unfailingly encouraged our work. Sandra Thompson and Mike Rechtienne were responsible for our first professional collaboration as a couple, bringing together insights from medicine and anthropology for global healthcare solutions. More recently, Terry Young has championed our combined expertise as part of his firm's intelligence reports and cultural briefings. In addition, we wish to acknowledge the contributions of Dr. Barbara Sahakian, Dr. Justin Roberts, Professor Martin Gibala, the incomparable dancer Michelle Dorrance, Dr. Lilianne Mujica-Parodi, Dr. Juan Manuel Antunez, Lama Yeshe, and Bodhicitta Chandigarh for in-depth discussions about their transformative work.

And now to matters of the heart. The love and support of our parents, Admiral Kirpal Singh and Manjit Kirpal Singh, sustained us throughout the writing of this book. We are grateful to our children Kirsty, Sophie, and Sahil. Indeed, all our cherished family members, crisscrossed across continents, especially my twin, Satpal, and siblings Neera, Prabha, Kamal, and Navpreet, have offered unfailing encouragement. After months of seclusion, an intense period when days and nights merged in writing this book, Devon MacEachron appeared as our angel of light with an energizing early reading of the manuscript. Time and again, we relied on Susan Hanna-Wicht, Libby Parella, and Daniel MacEachron for their invaluable insight. And on the occasions when we most needed it, this book has also benefited from the advice and buoyant humor of friends, among them (in alphabetical order) Claudine Giacchetti, Annalie Killian, Eiko and Tim McGregor, Tonia Pankopf, Punam Rai, Jean and Larry Shaw, Frederica Singh, Paola Porta and Teji Singh, Kermene Todywala, and Goolie Warburton.

Dr. Maclaren expresses gratitude to all the students and colleagues who have helped him to better understand the human condition and to his wife, Sunita Singh Maclaren, who did most of the heavy lifting for this book.

NOTES

Introduction

1. S. Pennazio, "Homeostasis: A History of Biology," *Rivista di Biologia* 102(2) (May–August 2009): 253–271.
2. Varman T. Samuel and Gerald I. Shulman, "Integrating Mechanisms for Insulin Resistance: Common Threads and Missing Links," *Cell* 148(5) (March 2, 2012): 852–871.
3. L. H. Lumey et al., "Prenatal Famine and Adult Health," *Annual Review of Public Health* 32 (2011): 237–262.
4. Stephanie Kullmann et al., "Brain Insulin Sensitivity Is Linked to Adiposity and Body Fat Distribution," *Nature Communications* 11 (2020): 1841.
5. "Global Statistics on Diabetes," Comment by Eberhard Standl, Forschergruppe Diabetes eV at Munich Helmholtz Centre, Germany for the EAPC Diabetes and CVD Educational Programme; European Society for Diabetes. April 2019.
6. Christopher A. Taylor, "Deaths from Alzheimer's Disease—United States, 1999–2014," *CDC Weekly* 66(20) (May 26, 2017): 521–526.
7. Guifen Xu et al., "Maternal Diabetes and the Risk of Autism Spectrum Disorders in the Offspring: A Systematic Review and Meta-Analysis," *Journal of Autism and Developmental Disorders* 44(4) (2014): 766–775.
8. N. K. Maclaren, S. Huang, and J. Fogh, "Antibody to Cultured Human Insulinoma Cells in Insulin-Independent Diabetes," *Lancet* 1 (1975): 997–999.
9. S. Huang and N. K. Maclaren, "Juvenile Diabetes: A Disease of Autoaggression," *Science* 192 (1976): 64–66.
10. M. Atkinson and N. K. Maclaren, "The Pathogenesis of Insulin Dependent Diabetes Mellitus," *New England Journal of Medicine* 331(21) (1994): 1428–1436.
11. M. A. Atkinson and N. K. Maclaren, "What Causes Diabetes?" *Scientific American* 262(7) (1990): 61–71.
12. W. Riley, N. K. Maclaren, J. Krischer, R. Spillar, J. Silverstein, D. Schatz, S. Shah, C. Vadheim, and J. Rotter, "A Prospective Study of the Development of Diabetes

in Relatives of Patients with Insulin Dependent Diabetes," *New England Journal of Medicine* 323 (1990): 1167–1172.

13. D. Schatz, J. Krischer, G. Horne, W. Riley, R. Spillar, J. Silverstein, W. Winter, A. Muir, D. Derovanesian, S. Shah, J. Malone, and N. K. Maclaren, "Islet Cell Antibodies Predict Insulin Dependent Diabetes in U.S. School Age Children as Powerfully as in Unaffected Relatives," *Journal of Clinical Investigation* 93 (1994): 2403–2407.

14. J. Silverstein, N. K. Maclaren, W. Riley, R. Spillar, D. Radjenovic, and S. Johnson, "Immunosuppression with Azathioprine and Prednisone in Recent-Onset Insulin-Dependent Diabetes Mellitus," *New England Journal of Medicine* 319(10) (1988): 599–604.

15. S. Ten and N. K. Maclaren, "Insulin Resistance Syndrome in Children," *Journal of Endocrinology and Metabolism* 89(6) (2004): 2526–2539.

16. Mateo Spinelli et al., "Brain Insulin Resistance and Hippocampal Plasticity: Mechanisms and Biomarkers of Cognitive Decline," *Frontiers in Neuroscience*, July 31, 2019, https://doi.org/10.3389/fnins.2019.00788.

17. Kristi A. Clark et al., "Dietary Fructose Intake and Hippocampal Structure and Connectivity during Childhood," *Nutrients* 12 (2020): 909; Geert Jan Biessels, "Hippocampal Insulin Resistance and Cognitive Dysfunction," *Nature* 16(11) (November 2015): 660–671.

18. Clifford Geertz, *The Interpretation of Cultures* (New York: Basic Books, 1973), 5.

Chapter 1. The Metabolic Matrix

1. Karen Hunger Parshall, *James Joseph Sylvester: Jewish Mathematician in a Victorian World* (Baltimore: Johns Hopkins University Press, 2006), 102.

2. Julie E. Flood-Obbagy and Barbara J. Rolls, "The Effect of Fruit in Different Forms on Energy Intake and Satiety at a Meal," *Appetite* 52(2) (2009): 416–422.

3. Marie Amitani, Akihiro Asakawa, et al., "The Role of Leptin in the Control of Insulin-Glucose Axis," *Frontiers in Neuroscience*, April 8, 2013, https://doi.org/10.3389/fnins.2013.00051.

4. Maria Foti and Massimo Locati, eds., *Cytokine Effector Functions in Tissues* (Cambridge, MA: Academic Press, 2017), 5.

5. Noureddine Benkeblia, ed., *Polysaccharides: Natural Fibers in Food and Nutrition* (Boca Raton, FL.: CRC Press, 2014), 261.

6. Lyna Kamintsky et al., "Blood-Brain Barrier Imaging as a Potential Biomarker for Bipolar Disorder Progression," *NeuroImage: Clinical* 26 (2020): 102049.

7. Sushmita Pamidi and Esra Tasali, "Obstructive Sleep Apnea and Type 2 Diabetes: Is There a Link?" *Frontiers in Neurology* 3 (2012): 126.

8. J. M. Fernandez-Real, M. Pugeat, M. Grasa, et al., "Serum Corticosteroid-Binding Globulin Concentration and Insulin Resistance Syndrome: A Population Study," *Journal of Clinical Endocrinology and Metabolism* 87(10) (2002): 4686–4690.

Chapter 2. Your Metabolism's Personality

1. Claude Bernard, *Introduction to the Study of Scientific Medicine*, translated by Henry Copley Greene (Henry Schuman, Inc., 1949).
2. L. Mujica-Parodi, A. Amgalan, S. Sultan, et al., "Diet Modifies Brain Network Stability, a Biomarker for Brain Aging, in Young Adults," *Proceedings of the National Academy of Sciences* 117(11) (2020): 6170–6177.
3. Anny H. Xiang et al., "Maternal Type 1 Diabetes and Risk of Autism in Offspring," *JAMA* 320 (2018): 89–91.

Chapter 3. Genetic Legacy: The Mischievous Messengers Lurking in Family Trees

1. Stephen O'Rahilly and I. Sadaf Farooqi, "Human Obesity: A Heritable Neurobehavioral Disorder That Is Highly Sensitive to Environmental Conditions," *Diabetes* 57(11) (2008): 2905–2910.
2. Deniz Atalayer et al., "Ghrelin and Eating Disorders," *Progress in Neuro-Psychopharmacology & Biological Psychiatry*, 40 (January 2013): 70–82.
3. S. H. Kim, "Measurement of Insulin Action: A Tribute to Sir Harold Himsworth," *Diabetic Medicine* 28 (2011): 1487–1493.
4. "NIH Study Shows How Insulin Stimulates Fat Cells to Take in Glucose," NIH news release, September 7, 2010, https://www.nih.gov/news-events/news-releases/nih-study-shows-how-insulin-stimulates-fat-cells-take-glucose.
5. Gibran Hemani et al., "Inference of the Genetic Architecture Underlying BMI and Height with the Use of 20,240 Sibling Pairs," *American Journal of Human Genetics* 93 (2013): 865–875.
6. "A Century of Trends in Adult Human Height," eLife, NCD Risk Factor Collaboration, July 26, 2016, eLife 2016; 5:e13410; DOI: 10.7554/eLife.13410.
7. Jenny van Dongen, Gonneke Willemsen, Wei-Min Chen, et al., "Heritability of Metabolic Syndrome Traits in a Large Population-Based Sample," *Journal of Lipid Research* 54 (2013): 2914–2923.
8. R. Arlen Price and Irving I. Gottesman, "Body Fat in Identical Twins Reared Apart: Roles for Genes and Environment," *Behavior Genetics* 21 (1991): 1–7.
9. Jihoon E. Joo et al., "Heritable DNA Methylation Marks Associated with Susceptibility to Breast Cancer," *Nature Communications* 9 (2018): 867.
10. Stephen B. Baylin and Peter A. Jones, "Epigenetic Determinants of Cancer," *Cold Spring Harbor Perspectives in Biology* 8(9) (2016): a019505.

11. Tatjana Buklijas, "Food, Growth, and Time: Elsie Widdowson's and Robert McCance's Research into Prenatal and Early Postnatal Growth," *Studies in History and Philosophy of Biological and Biomedical Sciences* Part B (2013), doi: 10.1016/j.shpsc.2013.12.001.

12. Kara Calkins and Sherin U. Devaskar, "Fetal Origins of Adult Disease," *Current Problems in Pediatric and Adolescent Health Care* 40(6) (2011): 158–176.

13. Lu Chen et al., "Identifying and Interpreting Apparent Neanderthal Ancestry in African Individuals," *Cell* 180(4) (2020): 677–687.

14. Robert G. Nelson, "Changing Course of Diabetic Nephropathy in the Pima Indians," *Diabetes Research and Clinical Practice* 82 (Suppl. 1) (2008): S10–S14.

15. Leslie O. Schulz and Lisa S. Chaudhari, "High-Risk Populations: The Pimas of Arizona and Mexico," *Current Obesity Reports* 4(1) (2015): 92–98.

16. James J. DiNicolantonio and James O'Keefe, "Markedly Increased Intake of Refined Carbohydrates and Sugar Is Associated with the Rise of Coronary Heart Disease and Diabetes among the Alaskan Inuit," *Open Heart* 2017; 4:e000673. doi: 10.1136/openhrt-2017-000673.

17. T. K. Young et al., "Prevalence of Obesity and Its Metabolic Correlates among the Circumpolar Inuit in 3 Countries," *American Journal of Public Health* 97(4) (2007): 691–695.

18. Sadaf Farooqi and Stephen O'Rahilly, "The Genetics of Obesity in Humans," Endotext, December 2017, https://www.ncbi.nlm.nih.gov/books/NBK279064/.

19. Albert J. Stunkard, Thorkild I. A. Sørensen, et al., "An Adoption Study of Human Obesity," *New England Journal of Medicine* 314 (1986): 193–198.

20. C. Willyard, "Heritability: The Family Roots of Excess Weight," *Nature* 508 (2014): S58–S60.

21. Hermine H. M. Maes, Michael C. Neale, and Lindon J. Eaves, "Genetic and Environmental Factors in Relative Body Weight and Human Adiposity," *Behavior Genetics* 27(4) (1997): 325–351.

22. T. W. Teasdale, T. I. Sørensen, and A. J. Stunkard, "Genetic and Early Environmental Components in Sociodemographic Influences on Adult Body Fatness," *British Medical Journal* 300 (1990): 1615–1618.

23. Sara Hiom, "A Tribute to Professor Jane Wardle," Cancer Research UK, October 23, 2015, https://scienceblog.cancerresearchuk.org/2015/10/23/professor-jane-wardle-30101950-20102015/.

24. Claire M. A. Haworth, Robert Plomin, Susan Carnell, and Jane Wardle. "Childhood Obesity: Genetic and Environmental Overlap with Normal-Range BMI," *Obesity* 16 (2008): 1585–1590.

25. James V. Neel, "The 'Thrifty Genotype' in 1998," *Nutrition Reviews* 57 (1999): 2–9.

26. *Journal of Inborn Errors of Metabolism and Screening;* Gilbert Thompson, *Pioneers of Medicine without a Nobel Prize* (London: Imperial College Press, 2014); Marisha Agana and Julia Frueh, "Common Metabolic Disorder (Inborn Errors of Metabolism) Concerns in Primary Care Practice" *Annals of Translational Medicine* 6(24) (2018): 469.

Chapter 4. Nutritional Profiles: Food, Culture, and Identity

1. Nancy J. Turner, *Food Plants of Coastal First Peoples* (Victoria: Royal British Columbia Museum, 1995), 17.

2. Richard W. Wrangham, *Catching Fire: How Cooking Made Us Human* (New York: Basic Books, 2010).

3. "High Blood Sugar Causes Brain Changes That Raise Depression Risk," Endocrine Society, *Science Daily*, June 2014, https://www.sciencedaily.com/releases/2014/06/140623092011.htm.

4. Birgit Wassermann et al., "An Apple a Day: Which Bacteria Do We Eat with Organic and Conventional Apples?" *Frontiers in Microbiology*, July 24, 2019, https://doi.org/10.3389/fmicb.2019.01629.

5. Leah E. Cahill et al., "Prospective Study of Breakfast Eating and Incident Coronary Heart Disease in a Cohort of Male US Health Professionals," *Circulation* 128(4) (2013): 337–343.

6. T. Aung, J. Halsey, and D. Kromhout, "Associations of Omega-3 Fatty Acids Supplement Use with Cardiovascular Disease Risks," *JAMA* 3(3) (2018): 225–233.

7. Fernando Gómez-Pinilla, "Brain Foods: The Effects of Nutrients on Brain Function," *Nature Reviews Neuroscience* 9(7) (2008): 568–578.

8. Sara Ipatenco, "The Average Sugar in a Smoothie," SFGate, December 6, 2018, https://healthyeating.sfgate.com/average-sugar-smoothie-12271.html.

9. Julia Flood-Obbagy and Barbara Rolls, "The Effect of Fruit in Different Forms on Energy Intake and Satiety at a Meal," *Appetite* 52(2) (2009): 416–422.

10. Hélène Labouré et al., "Behavioral, Plasma, and Calorimetric Changes Related to Food Texture Modification in Men," *American Journal of Physiology Regulatory, Integrative, and Comparative Physiology* 282 (2002): R1501–R1511.

11. Robert A. Bye Jr. and Edelmira Linares, "Mexican Market Plants of the 16th Century," *Journal of Ethnobiology* 10(2) (1990):151–168.

12. T. S. Eliot, *Notes towards the Definition of Culture* (New York: Harcourt Brace and Company, 1949), 27.

13. S. C. Ahuja and Uma Ahuja, "Rice in the Soul and Cultural Life of a People," in *Rice: Origin, Antiquity, and History,* edited by S. D. Sharma (Boca Raton, FL: CRC Press, 2010).

14. Nazanin Abbaspour et al. "Review on Iron and Its Importance for Human Health," *Journal of Research in the Medical Sciences* 19(2) (2014): 164–174.

15. T. Aung, J. Halsey, and D. Kromhout, "Associations of Omega-3 Fatty Acids Supplement Use with Cardiovascular Disease Risks," *JAMA* 3(3) (2018): 225–233.

Chapter 5. Hunger: Signals That Fine-Tune the Appetite

1. "Dr. John Eng's Research Found That the Saliva of the Gila Monster Contains a Hormone That Treats Diabetes Better than Any Other Medicine," Diabetes in Control, September 18, 2007, http://www.diabetesincontrol.com/dr-john-engs-research-found-that-the-saliva-of-the-gila-monster-contains-a-hormone-that-treats-diabetes-better-than-any-other-medicine/.

2. Andrew Pollack, "Lizard Linked Therapy Has Roots in the Bronx," *New York Times*, September 21, 2002.

3. Michael Gejl, "In Alzheimer's Disease, 6-Month Treatment with GLP-1 Analog Prevents Decline of Brain Glucose Metabolism: Randomized, Placebo-Controlled, Double-Blind Clinical Trial," *Frontiers of Aging Neuroscience* 8 (2016): 108.

4. Ernest Hemingway, *A Moveable Feast* (Scribner, 1972), 71.

5. Carlos A. Monteiro, "Ultra-Processed Foods: What They Are and How to Identify Them," *Public Health Nutrition* 22(5) (2019): 936–941.

6. Duke Stanford podcast, "The Leading Voice on Food," Episode 24, March 26, 2019.

7. Shan Luo, "Differential Effects of Fructose versus Glucose on Brain and Appetitive Responses to Food Cues and Decisions for Food Rewards," *Proceedings of the National Academy of Science USA* 112(20) (2015): 6509–6514.

8. Nicola J. Buckland, "Women with a Low-Satiety Phenotype Show Impaired Appetite Control and Greater Resistance to Weight Loss," *British Journal of Nutrition* 122 (2019): 951–959.

9. Elizabeth J. Reverri, "Assessing Beans as a Source of Intrinsic Fiber on Satiety in Men and Women with Metabolic Syndrome," *Appetite* 118 (2017): 75–81.

10. Nuno Casanova, John Blundell, et al., "Biopsychology of Human Appetite—Understanding the Excitatory and Inhibitory Mechanisms of Homeostatic Control," *Physiology* 12 (2019): 33–38.

11. D. Dolinoy, D. Huma, and R. Jirtle, "Maternal Nutrient Supplementation Counteracts Bisphenol A Induced DNA Hypomethylation in Early Development," *Proceedings of the National Academy of Sciences* 104(32) (2007): 13056–13061.

12. Catherine Gibbons, Mark Hopkins, Kristine Beaulieu, Pauline Oustric, and John E. Blundell, "Issues in Measuring and Interpreting Human Appetite (Satiety/Satiation) and Its Contribution to Obesity," *Obesity Reports*, April 2019.

13. *The Comedy of Errors*, William Shakespeare, Act I, Scene V.

14. Hannah M. Bayer and Paul W. Glimcher, "Midbrain Dopamine Neurons Encode a Quantitative Reward Prediction Error Signal," *Neuron* 47 (2005): 129–141.

15. Nora D. Volkow, "Dopamine in Drug Abuse and Addiction," *Archives of Neurology* 64(11) (2007): 1575–1579.

16. L. C. Daws, M. J. Avison, and S. D. Robertson, "Insulin Signaling and Addiction," *Neuropharmacology* 61(7) (2011): 1123–1128.

17. Mirre Viskaal-van Dongen et al., "Eating Rate of Commonly Consumed Foods Promotes Food and Energy Intake," *Appetite* 56(1) (2011): 25–31.

18. Hayley Syrad, "Meal Size Is a Critical Driver of Weight Gain in Early Childhood," *Nature, Scientific Reports* 6 (2016): 28368.

19. Anna Fogel et al., "Faster Eating Rates Are Associated with Higher Energy Intakes," *British Journal of Nutrition* 117 (2017): 1042–1051.

20. Chul-Kyoo Kim, Hyun-Jin Kim, Hae-Kyung Chung, and Dayeon Shin, "Eating Alone Is Differentially Associated with the Risk of Metabolic Syndrome in Korean Men and Women," *Environmental Research and Public Health*, 15 (2018): 1020.

Chapter 6. Gut Reaction: The Power of the Microbiome

1. Ambrose Bierce, "Esophagus," in *The Devil's Dictionary* (Athens, GA: University of Georgia Press).

2. Luba Vikhanski, *Immunity: How Elie Metchnikoff Changed the Course of Modern Medicine* (Chicago: Chicago Review Press, 2016).

3. D. J. Bibel, "Elie Metchnikoff's Bacillus of Long Life," *ASM News* 54 (1988): 661–665.

4. Niall Hyland and Catherine Stanton, *The Gut-Brain Axis: Dietary, Probiotic, and Prebiotic Interventions on the Microbiota* (London: Academic Press, 2016), 1.

5. Karen E. Nelson, *Metagenics of the Human Body* (New York: Springer, 2010): viii.

6. V. Ahlqvist, M. Persson, C. Magnusson, and D. Berglind, "Elective and Nonelective Cesarean Section and Obesity among Young Adult Male Offspring: A Swedish Population Based Cohort," *PLOS Medicine* 2019 16(12), e1002996.

7. N. T. Mueller, E. Bakacs, J. Combellick, Z. Grigoryan, and M. G. Dominguez-Bello, "The Infant Microbiome Development: Mom Matters," *Trends in Molecular Medicine* 21(2) (2015): 109–117.

8. A. Kukreja and N. Maclaren, "NKT Cells and Type-1 Diabetes and the 'Hygiene Hypothesis' to Explain the Rising Incidence Rates," *Diabetes Technology & Therapeutics* 4(3) (2002): 323–333.

9. J. J. Faith, J. L. Guruge, M. Charbonneau, S. Subramanian, H. Seedorf, A. L. Goodman, J. C. Clemente, R. Knight, A. C. Heath, R. L. Leibel, M. Rosenbaum,

and J. I. Gordon, "The Long-Term Stability of the Human Gut Microbiota," *Science* 341(6141) (2013):1237439.

10. E. Le Chatelier, T. Nielsen, J. Qin, E. Prifti, F. Hildebrand, G. Falony, et al., "Richness of Human Gut Microbiome Correlates with Metabolic Markers," *Nature* 500(7464) (2013): 541–546.

11. Megan Clapp, "The Gut's Effect on Mental Health-Brain Axis," *Clinical Practice* 7(4) (2017): 987.

12. Rachel Hajar, "The Air of History (Part V) Ibn Sina (Avicenna): The Great Physician and Philosopher," *Heart Views* 14(4) (2013): 196–201.

13. A. Sarkar and P. W. Burnet, "Psychobiotics and the Manipulation of Bacteria-Gut-Brain Signals," *Trends in Neuroscience* 39 (2016): 763–781.

14. Ed Yong, *I Contain Multitudes* (New York: Ecco, 2016): 223.

15. J. R. Kelly, A. P. Allen, A. Temko, W. Hutch, P. J. Kennedy, N. Farid, E. Murphy, G. Boylan, J. Bienenstock, J. F. Cryan, G. Clarke, and T. G. Dinan, "Lost in translation? The Potential Psychobiotic Lactobacillus Rhamnosus (Jb-1) Fails to Modulate Stress or Cognitive Performance in Healthy Male Subjects," *Brain, Behavior, and Immunity* 61 (2017): 50–59.

16. A. R. Romijn, J. J. Rucklidge, R. G. Kuijer, and C. Frampton, "A Double-Blind, Randomized, Placebo-Controlled Trial of Lactobacillus Helveticus and Bifidobacterium Longum for the Symptoms of Depression," *Australian and New Zealand Journal of Psychiatry* 51 (2017): 810–821.

17. S. Arslanoglu, G. E. Moro, and G. Boehm, "Early Supplementation of Prebiotic Oligosaccharides Protects Formula-Fed Infants against Infections during the First 6 Months of Life," *Journal of Nutrition* 137(11) (2007): 2420–2424.

18. S. Arslanoglu, G. E. Moro, J. Schmitt, L. Tandoi, S. Rizzardi, and G. Boehm, "Early Dietary Intervention with a Mixture of Prebiotic Oligosaccharides Reduces the Incidence of Allergic Manifestations and Infections during the First Two Years of Life," *Journal of Nutrition* 138(6) (2008): 1091–1095.

19. P. D. Cani, E. Lecourt, E. M. Dewulf, F. M. Sohet, B. D. Pachikian, D. Naslain, F. De Backer, A. M. Neyrinck, and N. M. Delzenne, "Gut Microbiota Fermentation of Prebiotics Increases Satietogenic and Incretin Gut Peptide Production with Consequences for Appetite Sensation and Glucose Response after a Meal," *American Journal of Clinical Nutrition* 90(5) (2009):1236–1243.

20. K. R. Freeland, C. Wilson, and T. M. Wolever, "Adaptation of Colonic Fermentation and Glucagon-Like Peptide-1 Secretion with Increased Wheat Fiber Intake for 1 Year in Hyper Insulinemic Human Subjects," *British Journal of Nutrition* 103 (2010): 82–90.

21. W. Riley, P. Toskes, N. Maclaren, and J. H. Silverstein, "Predictive Value of Gastric Parietal Cell Autoantibodies as a Marker for Gastric and Hematological Abnormalities Associated with Insulin Dependent Diabetes," *Diabetes* 31 (1982): 1051–1055.

22. Jim Powell, "Alexis de Tocqueville: How People Gain Liberty and Lose It," Foundation for Economic Education, July 1996, https://fee.org/articles/alexis-de -tocqueville-how-people-gain-liberty-and-lose-it/.

23. Graham Farmelo, *The Strangest Man* (New York: Basic Books, 2009), 1.

Chapter 7. Fat Cells: Exquisitely Designed Hubs of Energy?

1. William Shakespeare, *Romeo and Juliet*, Act 1, Scene 1.

2. O. H. Wolff and June K. Lloyd, "Childhood Excess Weight," *Proceedings of Nutritional Society* (32)3 (1973): 195–198.

3. Gordon C Weir, J. Larry Jameson, and Leslie J. De Groot, *Endocrinology Adult and Pediatric: Diabetes Mellitus and Obesity*, Chap. 11 (Philadelphia: Saunders, 2010), 162.

4. Min Jae Kang, "The Adiposity Rebound in the 21st Century Children," *Korean Journal of Pediatrics* 61(12) (2018): 375–380.

5. Dimitrius Vlachakis, *Adipocyte Viability and LDH* (Luton, Bedfordshire, UK: Bedfordshire University, 2007), 8.

6. Nancy Costello, "Women Are Better Able than Men to Survive Calamity, Research Finds," *Los Angeles Times,* January 12, 1992.

7. Donald K. Grayson, "Donner Party Deaths: A Demographic Assessment," *Journal of Anthropological Research* 46(3) (1990): 223–242.

8. R. P. Donahue, "Central Obesity and Coronary Heart Disease in Men," *Lancet* 1(8537) (1987): 821–824.

9. Kirsty Spalding, "Dynamics of Fat Cell Turonover in Humans" *Nature* 453(7196): 783–787.

10. Marco Arrese, "The Liver in Poetry: Neruda's 'Ode to the Liver,'" *Liver International* 27(7) (2008): 901–905, https://doi.org/10.1111/j.1478-3231.2008.01814.x.

11. George Fodor, "Primary Prevention of CVD: Treating Dyslipidemia," *American Family Physician* 83(10) (2011): 1207–1208.

12. Prakash Deedwania, *Prevention of Cardiovascular Disease* (Philadelphia: Saunders, 2011), 127.

13. Mathias J. Betz, "Human Brown Adipose Tissue: What We Have Learned So Far," *Diabetes* 64(7) (2015): 2352–2360.

14. "Role of miRNAs in Brown and White Adipose Tissue Differentiation and Function," MIRBATWAT, European Research Council, February 2014.

Chapter 8. Energy: Speed, Strength, Movement, and Agility

1. Deborah Muoio, "Metabolic Inflexibility: When Mitochondrial Indecision Leads to Metabolic Gridlock," *Cell* 159(6) (2014): 1253–1262.

2. Lykke Sylow, "Exercise-Stimulated Glucose Uptake—Regulation and Implications for Glycemic Control," *National Review of Endocrinology* 13(3) (2017): 133–148.

3. Gary D. Foster and Brian G. McGuckin, "Estimating Resting Energy Expenditure in Obesity," *Obesity Research* 9 (2001): 367S–372S.

4. J. Kerns, J. Guo, E. Fothergill, et al., "Increased Physical Activity Associated with Less Weight Regain Six Years after 'The Biggest Loser' Competition," *Obesity* 25 (2017): 1838–1849.

5. Vassilis Mougios, *Exercise Biochemistry* (Champaign, IL: Human Kinetics, 2019), 299.

6. W. Martin and M. Mentel, "The Origin of Mitochondria," *Nature Education* 3(9) (2010): 58.

7. Andrew J. Roger, "The Origin and Diversification of Mitochondria," *Current Biology* 27 (2017): R1177–R1192.

8. J. Langdahi and A. Frederson, "Mitochondrial Mutation in M324A>G Associated with Insulin Resistance in Non-Diabetic Carriers," *Endocrine Connections* 8(7) (2019): 529–837.

9. G. C. Conroy and H. Pontzer, *Reconstructing Human Origins: A Modern Synthesis*, 3rd ed. (New York: Norton, 2012).

10. Leslie C. Aiello, "Brains and Guts in Human Evolution: The Expensive Tissue Hypothesis," *Brazilian Journal of Genetics* 20(1) (1997), https://doi.org/10.1590/S0100-84551997000100023.

11. W. R. Leonard and M. L. Robertson, "Comparative Primate Energetics and Hominid Evolution," *American Journal of Physical Anthropology* 102 (1997): 265–281.

12. Karen Clippinger, *Dance Anatomy and Kinesiology*, 2nd edition (Champaign, IL: Human Kinetics, 2016), 33.

13. Brad J. Schonfeld, "Resistance Training Volume Enhances Muscle Hypertrophy but Not Strength in Trained Men," *Medicine & Science in Sports & Exercise* 51(1) (2019): 94–103.

14. Gerald Shulman, "The Role of Skeletal Muscle Insulin Resistance in the Pathogenesis of the Metabolic Syndrome," *Proceedings of the National Academy of Sciences* 104(31) (2007): 12587–12594.

15. Eric Bartholomae, "Reducing Glycemic Indicators with Moderate Intensity Stepping of Varied, Short Durations in People with Pre-Diabetes," *Journal of Sports Science and Medicine* 17 (2018): 680–685.

16. David A. Hood, "Mechanisms of Exercise-Induced Mitochondrial Biogenesis in Skeletal Muscle," *Applied Physiology, Nutrition, and Metabolism* 34 (2009): 465–472.

17. Robert McMurray, *Concepts in Fitness Programming* (Boca Raton, FL: CRC Press, 2019).

18. Martin P. Schwellnus, ed. *The Olympic Textbook of Medicine in Sports* (Oxford: Wiley-Blackwell, 2009), 94.

19. Kenneth Laws, *Physics and the Art of Dance: Understanding Movement* (New York: Oxford University Press, 2002).

20. C. Bouchard et al., "Familial Aggregation of VO(2max) Response to Exercise Training: Results from the HERITAGE Family Study," *Journal of Applied Physiology* 87(3) (1999):1003–1008.

21. Alfonso J. Cruz-Jentoft and Francesco Landi, "Sarcopenia," *Clinical Medicine* 14 (2) (2014): 183–186.

22. S.-J. Park, O. Gavilova, A. Brown, et al., "DNA-PK Promotes the Mitochondrial, Metabolic and Physical Decline that Occurs during Aging," *Cell Metabolism* 25(5) (2017): 1135–1148.

23. K. Stanford and L. Goodyear, "Exercise and Type-2 Diabetes: Molecular Mechanisms Regulating Glucose Uptake in Skeletal Muscle," *Advances in Physiology Education* 38(4) (2014): 308–314.

Chapter 9. Enriching Cognition: Thoughts, Mood, and Memory

1. Benjamin Scholl, "The Cortical Connection," *Nature* 518(7539) (2015): 306–307.

2. D. D. Clark and L. Sokoloff, "Circulation and Energy Metabolism of the Brain," in *Basic Neurochemistry: Molecular, Cellular and Medical Aspects*, edited by G. J. Siegel, B. W. Agranoff, R. W. Albers, S. K. Risher, and M. D. Uhler (Philadelphia: Lippincott, 1999), 637–670.

3. Daniel J. Siegel, *The Developing Mind: How Relationships and the Brain Interact to Shape Who We Are* (New York: Guilford Press, 2020), 4.

4. L. Mujica-Parodi, A. Amgalan, S. Sultan, et al., "Diet Modifies Brain Network Stability, a Biomarker for Brain Aging, in Young Adults," *Proceedings of the National Academy of Sciences* 117(11) (2020): 6170-6177 e.

5. Jessica Wright, "The Real Reasons Autism Rates Are Up in the U.S.," *Spectrum,* March 3, 2017.

6. "Data and Statistics on Autism Spectrum Disorder," Centers for Disease Control and Prevention, https://www.cdc.gov/ncbddd/autism/data.html.

7. "The State of Mental Health in America," Mental Health America, www.mhanational.org.

8. "Facts and Figures," Alzheimer's Association, www.alz.org.

9. Sophia Frangou, "Insulin Resistance: Genetic Associations with Depression and Cognition," *Experimental Neurology* 316 (2019): 20–26.

10. Michael L. Alosco and Robert A. Stern, *The Oxford Handbook of Cognitive Decline* (New York: Oxford University Press, 2019), 125.

11. "New Findings Could Improve Diagnosis, Treatment of Depression," *Berkeley News*, October 28, 2019.

12. Sandrine Ceurstemont, "Pinning Down Consciousness Could Improve Mental Health, Brain Disorder Treatments," *Horizon: EU Research and Innovation*, November 13, 2019.

13. Giorgi A. Ascoti, *Trees of the Brain, Roots of the Mind* (Boston: MIT Press, 2015).

14. Robert Lawrence Kuhn, "Brains, Minds, AI, God: Marvin Minsky Thought Like No One Else (Tribute)," March 4, 2016, https://www.space.com/32153-god-artificial-intelligence-and-the-passing-of-marvin-minsky.html.

15. John M. Freeman, "Epilepsy's Big Fat Answer," *Cerebrum* (2013), PMC3662214.

16. Susan A. Masino, *Ketogenic Diets and Metabolic Therapy* (New York: Oxford University Press, 2016), x.

17. Laura L. Ekblad et al., "Insulin Resistance Predicts Cognitive Decline: An 11-Year Follow-up of Nationally Representative Adult Population Sample," *Diabetes Care* 40 (2017): 751–758.

18. *Lancet Psychiatry* Editorial Volume 5, January 1, 2018.

19. Hannah Ritchie and Max Roser, "Mental Health," Our World in Data, April 2018, https://ourworldindata.org/mental-health.

20. E. Jane Costello, "The Great Smoky Mountains Study: Developmental Epidemiology in the Southeastern United States." *Social Psychiatry and Psychiatric Epidemiology* 51(5) (2016): 639–646.

21. Anne-Marie Mouly and Regina Sullivan, "Memory and Plasticity in the Olfactory System: From Infancy to Adulthood," in *The Neurobiology of Olfaction*, edited by L. Menini (Boca Raton, FL: CRC Press, 2015).

22. Marianna E. Hayiou-Thomas, "When Does Speech Sound Disorder Matter for Literacy? The Role of Disordered Speech Errors, Co-occurring Language Impairment and Family Risk of Dyslexia," *Journal of Child Psychology and Psychiatry* 58(2) (2017): 197–205.

23. Edith Bird LaFrance, "The Gifted/Dyslexic Child: Characterizing and Addressing Strengths and Weaknesses," *Annals of Dyslexia* 47 (1997): 163–182.

24. Katja Beesdo, "Anxiety and Anxiety Disorders in Children and Adolescents: Developmental Issues and Implications for DSM-V," *Psychiatric Clinics of North America* 32(3) (2009): 483–524.

25. Amelia Heathman, "Decoder: New Brain Training App Launched to Improve Concentration Skills and Attention Span," *Evening Standard*, January 21, 2019, https://

www.standard.co.uk/tech/decoder-brain-training-app-university-of-cambridge -a4044201.html.

26. Yael Natz, "Is There a Preferred Mode of Exercise for Cognition Enhancement in Older Age?" *Frontiers in Medicine,* March 29, 2019, https://doi.org/10.3389 /fmed.2019.00057.

27. M. Pappolla, L. Manchikanti, C. Andersen, et al., "Is Insulin Resistance the Cause of Fibromyalgia? A Preliminary Report," *PLOS ONE* 14(5) (2019): e0216079.

28. G. Hausman, U. Basu, M. Du, et al., "Intermuscular and Intramuscular Adipose Tissues, Bad vs. Good Adipose Tissues, *Adipocyte* 3 (2014): 4.

29. Moheb Constandi, *Neuroplasticity* (Boston: MIT Press, 2016). 5.

30. A. Negele et al., "Childhood Trauma and Its Relation to Chronic Depression in Adulthood," *Depression Research and Treatment*, https://doi.org/10.1155 /2015/650804.

31. Natalie Nanayakkara, "Depression and Diabetes Distress in Adults with Type 2 Diabetes: Results from the Australian National Diabetes Audit (ANDA) 2016," *Nature Scientific Reports* 8, Article 7846 (2018).

32. M. C. Austin et al., "Increased Corticotropin-Releasing Hormone Immunoreactivity in Monoamine-Containing Pontine Nuclei of Depressed Suicide Men," *Molecular Psychiatry* 8(3) (2003): 324–332.

33. Nir Barzilai et al., "Metformin as a Tool to Target Aging," *Cell Metabolism* 23 (2016): 1060–1065.

34. R. Tuligenga, A. Dugravot, A. Tabak, et al., "Midlife Type-2 Diabetes and Poor Glycemic Control as Risk Factors for Cognitive Decline in Early Old Age: A Post-hoc Analysis of the Whitehall II Cohort Study," *Lancet: Diabetes and Endocrinology* 2(3) (2014): 228–235.

35. Mark P. Mattson et al., "Intermittent Metabolic Switching, Neuroplasticity, and Brain Health," *Nature Reviews Neuroscience* 19 (2018): 81–94.

36. Andrew Octavian Sasmita, "Harnessing Neuroplasticity: Modern Approaches and Clinical Future," *International Journal of Neuroscience* 128(11) (2018): 1061– 1077.

37. Joyce Schaffer, "Neuroplasticity and Clinical Practice: Building Brain Power For Health," *Frontiers in Psychology* 7 (2016): 1118.

38. Richard J. Davidson and Bruce McEwen, "Social Influences on Neuroplasticity: Stress and Interventions to Promote Well-being," *Nature Neuroscience* 15(5) (2012): 689–695.

Chapter 10. Stress Responses: On Mental Resilience

1. Y. H. Song, E. L. Connor, A. Muir, J. X. She, B. Zorovich, D. Derovanesian, and N. Maclaren, "Autoantibody Epitope Mapping of the 21-Hydroxylase Antigen in Autoimmune Addison's Disease," *Journal of Clinical Endocrinology and Metabolism* 78(5) (1994): 1108–1112.

2. Siang Yong Tan, "Hans Selye (1907–1982): Founder of the Stress Theory," *Singapore Medical Journal* 59(4) (2018): 170–171.

3. Hans Selye, *The Stress of Life* (New York: McGraw-Hill, 1956), 4.

4. Mark Jackson, "The Pursuit of Happiness," *History of the Human Sciences* 25(5) (2012): 13–29.

5. Marci E. Gluck, "Stress Response and Binge Eating Disorder," *Appetite* 46 (2006): 26–30.

6. E. Oppenheimer, "Decreased Insulin Sensitivity in Prepubertal Girls with Premature Adrenarche and Acanthosis Nigricans," *Journal of Clinical Endocrinology and Metabolism* 80(2) (1995):614–618.

7. Ora Hirsch Pescovitz and Erica A. Eugster, *Pediatric Endocrinology* (Philadelphia: Lippincott, Williams, and Wilkins, 2004), 365.

8. J. R. Kaplan, S. B. Manuck, et al., "Social Stress and Atherosclerosis in Normocholesterolemic Monkeys," *Science* 220(4598) (1983): 733–735.

9. George Fink, ed., *Stress: Concepts, Cognition, Emotion, and Behavior* (Cambridge, MA: Academic Press, 2016), 117.

10. Geoffrey Canet, "Central Role of Glucocorticoid Receptors in Alzheimer's Disease and Depression," *Frontiers in Neuroscience* 12 (2018): 739.

11. C. Geelam, E. van Greevenbrook, W. van Rossum, et al., "Bcl1 Glucocorticoid Receptor Polymorphism Is Associated with Greater Body Fatness: The HOORN and CODAM Studies," *Journal of Clinical Endocrinology and Metabolism* (2013): E595–E599.

12. Tobias Stalder, "Cortisol in Hair and the Metabolic Syndrome," *Journal of Clinical Endocrinology and Metabolism* 98(6) (2013): 2573–2580.

13. R. Shweder, "America's Latest Export: A Stressed-Out World," *New York Times,* January 26, 1997.

14. S. Mechiel Korte, Jaap M. Koolhaas, John C. Wingfield, and Bruce S. McEwen, "The Darwinian Concept of Stress: Benefits of Allostasis and Costs of Allostatic Load and the Trade-Offs in Health and Disease," *Neuroscience and Biobehavioral Reviews* 29(1) (2005): 3–38.

15. Jon Kabat-Zinn, *Full Catastrophe Living*, 15th ann. ed. (New York: Random House, 2005), 235.

16. R. J. Daly, "Samuel Pepys and Post-Traumatic Stress Disorder," *British Journal of Psychiatry* 143(1) (1983): 64–68.

17. David G. Myers, *Exploring Psychology*, 8th ed. (New York: Worth Publishers, 2005), 408.

18. "Stress in America: Stress and Current Events." American Psychological Association, Stress in America Survey 2019, https://www.apa.org/news/press/releases/stress/2019/stress-america-2019.pdf.

19. Bruce S. McEwen and Huda Akil, "Revisiting the Stress Concept: Implications for Affective Disorders," *Journal of Neuroscience* 40(1) (2020): 12–21.

20. Gary W. Miller, "The Nature of Nurture: Refining the Definition of the Exposome," *Toxicological Studies* 137(1) (2014): 1–2.

21. Armin P. Moczek, "The Role of Developmental Plasticity in Evolutionary Innovation," *Proceedings of the Royal Society B* 278 (2011): 2705–2713.

22. Eun Joo Kim, "Stress Effects on the Hippocampus: A Critical Review," *Learning & Memory* 22(9) (2015): 411–416.

23. David Mischouloun, "Depression and Eating Disorders: Treatment and Course," *Journal of Affective Disorders* 130(3) (2011): 470–477.

24. Janet Tomiyama, "How and Why Weight Stigma Drives the Obesity 'Epidemic' and Harms Health," *BMC Medicine* (2018) 16: 123.

25. S. A. Richardson, N. Goodman, A. H. Hastorf, and S. M. Dornbusch, "Cultural Uniformity in Reaction to Physical Disabilities," *American Sociological Review* 26(2) (1961): 241–247.

26. Mary Himmelstein and A. Janet Tomiyama, "It's Not You, It's Me: Self-Perceptions, Antifat Attitudes, and Stereotyping of Obese Individuals," *Social Psychological and Personality Science* 6(7) (2015): 749–757.

27. A. F. Corning, A. J. Krumm, and L. A. Smitham, "Differential Social Comparison Processes in Women with and without Eating Disorder Symptoms," *Journal of Counseling Psychology* 53(3) (2006): 338–349.

28. John Beddington et al., "The Mental Wealth of Nations," *Nature* 455 (2008): 1057–1060.

29. Thomas J. Bouchard et al., "Sources of Human Psychological Differences, the Minnesota Study of Twins Reared Apart," *Science* 250 (1990): 223–228.

30. Ronald Purser, "The Myth of the Present Moment," *Mindfulness* 6 (2015): 680–686.

31. Marc Kaufman, "Meditation Gives the Brain a Charge," *Washington Post*, January 3, 2005.

Chapter 11. Sleep: Circadian Rhythm and Blues

1. Charles Nunn, "Sleep in a Comparative Context: Investigating How Human Sleep Differs from Sleep in Other Primates," *American Journal of Physical Anthropology* 166 (3) (2018): 601–612.

2. Takeshi Kanda, Takehiro Miyazaki, and Masashi Yanagisawa, "Imaging Sleep and Wakefulness," in *Make Life Visible*, edited by Y. Toyama, A. Miyawaki, M. Nakamura, and M. Jinzaki (Singapore: Springer, 2020), 169–178.

3. William H. Moorcraft, *Understanding Sleep and Dreaming* (New York: Springer, 2005): 42; Gregory Belenky et al., *The Effects of Sleep Deprivation on Performance during Continuous Combat Operations*, National Academy of Science (1994).

4. Walter B. Cannon, "Organization for Physiological Homeostasis," *Phsyiological Reviews* 9(3) (July 1929).

5. Jong Y. Lee, "A Tribute to Franz Halberg," *Hypertension* 66 (2015): 1090–1092.

6. Dr. Maiken Nedergaard, "How Sleep Clears the Brain," NIH news releases, NIH Research, October 28, 2013, https://www.nih.gov/news-events/news-releases/brain-may-flush-out-toxins-during-sleep.

7. Patrick McNamara, *Dreams and Visions: How Religious Ideas Emerge in Sleep and Dreams* (Santa Barbara, CA: Praeger, 2016), 24.

8. D. H. Lawrence, *The Fox/The Captain's Doll/The Ladybird* (New York: Penguin Classics, 2006).

9. American Thoracic Society, "Sleeping Less Linked to Weight Gain," Science Daily, May 29, 2006, https://www.sciencedaily.com/releases/2006/05/060529082903.htm.

10. Samuel Taylor Coleridge, "The Pains of Sleep," *Christabel*, 2nd edition (London: William Bulmer, 1816).

11. Anna Wirz-Justice, "Perspectives in Affective Disorders: Clocks and Sleep," *European Journal of Neuroscience* 51 (2020): 346–365.

12. Venkatramanujan Srinivasan, *Melatonin Therapeutic Value and Neuroprotection* (Boca Raton, FL: CRC Press, 2014), 290.

13. Jameson et al., *Endocrinology* (2010): 214.

14. Jong Y. Lee et al., "A Tribute to Franz Halberg," *Hypertension* 66 (2015): 1090–1092.

15. Paul Huebener et al., *Time, Globalization, and Human Experience* (Abingdon, UK: Routledge, 2016).

16. Dirk Jan Stenvers et al., "Circadian Clocks and Insulin Resistance," *Nature Review: Endocrinology* 15 (2019): 75–89.

17. Ahmed S. BaHammam, Wael Almestehi, et al., "Distribution of Chronotypes in a Large Sample of Young Adult Saudis," *Annals of Saudi Medicine* 31(2) (2011): 182–186.

18. Abbas Smiley et al., "Mechanisms of Association of Sleep and Metabolic Syndrome," *Journal of Medical and Clinical Research & Review* 3 (2019): 1–9.

19. M. S. Albreiki, B. Middleton, and S. M. Hampton, "A Single Night Light Exposure Acutely Alters Hormonal and Metabolic Responses in Healthy Participants," *Endocrine Connect* 6 (2017): 100–110.

20. Lijuan Xiu, Mirjam Ekstedt, et al., "Sleep and Adiposity in Children from 2 to 6 Years of Age," *Pediatrics* 145 (2020): e20191420.

21. Juan Manuel Antunez, "Circadian Typology Is Related to Emotion Regulation, Metacognitive Beliefs, and Assertiveness in Healthy Adults," *PLOS ONE,* March 2020.

22. Dieter Riemann et al., "Sleep, Insomnia, and Depression," *Neuropsychopharmacology* 45(1) (2020): 74–89.

23. John W. Winkelman et al., "Sleep and Neurpsychiatric Illness," *Neuropsychopharmacology* 45 (2020): 1–2.

Chapter 12. Hormone Imbalances: A Few Cases of False Alarms

1. R. G. Jung, T. Simard, et al., "Role of Plasminogen Activator Inhibitor-1 in Coronary Pathophysiology," *Thrombosis Research* 164 (2018): 54–62.

2. J. M. Fernandez-Real, M. Pugeat, M. Grasa, et al., "Serum Corticosteroid-Binding Globulin Concentration and Insulin Resistance Syndrome: A Population Study," *Journal of Clinical Endocrinology and Metabolism* 87(10) (2002): 4686–4690.

3. B. Daka, T. Rosen, Per-Anders Jansson, et al., "Inverse Association between Serum Insulin and Sex Hormone-Binding Globulin in a Population Survey in Sweden," *Endocrine Connect* 2(1) (2013): 18–22.

4. Michael R. Laurent, "Sex Hormone-Binding Globulin Regulation of Androgen Bioactivity in Vivo: Validation of the Free Hormone Hypothesis," *Scientific Reports* 6 (2016): 35539.

5. "Frida and the Miscarriage," lithograph, 1932.

6. Adi Dastur et al., "Irving Stein, Michael Leventhal, and a Slice of Endocrine History," *Journal of Obstetrics and Gynecology India* 60(2) (2010): 121–122.

7. Michael T. Sheehan, "Polycystic Ovarian Syndrome: Diagnosis and Management," *Clinical Medicine and Research* 2(1) (2004): 13–27.

INDEX

ABOUT THE AUTHORS

Dr. Noel Maclaren is an award-winning pioneer in endocrinology and the metabolism who practices in New York. He is a professor of pediatrics at the Weill College of Medicine of Cornell University and the co-founder of MetaKura. In his practice, Dr. Maclaren specializes in internal medicine, endocrinology, and metabolism in adults, children, and pregnant women. He has been listed multiple times on the annual "Best Doctors in America" by The Best Doctors Group at Harvard University. His numerous other awards include the Juvenile Diabetes Foundation International Award, David Rumbough Scientific Award, the International Research Canadian Diabetes Association/Connaught Novo Nordisk Award, Mary Jane Kugel Award, and his research has been funded by multiple NIH grants.

Sunita Singh Maclaren is the cofounder and CEO of MetaKura's digital platform and its Metabolism Innovation Lab. She also personally coaches individuals. Prior to this, she was founder of World Wise, a cultural advisory firm known for its tailored, local knowledge-based solutions for the global challenges faced by governmental agencies and nonprofits. Her expertise in representing the values and priorities of local communities in over thirty countries, including those in West Africa, the Russian Far East, and South East Asia, has been sought by the world's leading corporations. In rural India and China, she has worked in the area of medical anthropology. She continues to study the relationships between cultural and social health behavior, as well as people's beliefs about their metabolism.